THE INTERDISCIPLINARY HEALTH CARE TEAM

A Handbook

Alex J. Ducanis,
University of Pittsburgh

and

Anne K. Golin,
University of Pittsburgh

Aspen Systems Corporation
Germantown, Maryland
London, England
1979

Library of Congress Cataloging in Publication Data

Ducanis, Alex J.
The interdisciplinary health care team.

Includes bibliographical references and index.

1. Health care teams.
I. Golin, Anne K., joint author.   II Title.
R729.5.H4D83   610.69'6   79-21028
ISBN 0-89443-167-6

Library of Congress Catalog Card Number: 79-21028
ISBN: 0-89443-167-6

Printed in the United States of America

2 3 4 5

To our parents –

Frances Harrison Keefe
James L. Keefe
Virginia Vowinkel Ducanis
Alexander J. Ducanis

Table of Contents

Preface

This book has grown from a number of experiences over the past few years, both in the health fields and in education. Most directly, it is the outcome of a course in the Interdisciplinary Team which we designed and taught in the University of Pittsburgh's School of Health Related Professions.

The topic changed somewhat as the book developed. Initially the focus was on how teams make decisions about individuals. As the work progressed it became apparent that the body of empirical research dealing directly with teamwork was small and that additional work was needed. Much of what has been written about teams falls into the category of anecdotal material lauding the team approach, or experiential descriptions of "successful" and "unsuccessful" teams. While such efforts are useful in defining the area to be explored, they fall short when trying to explain team function or pointing to avenues of improving team effectiveness.

A second factor soon apparent was that there was little agreement on the definition of "professional teamwork." Authors idiosyncratically use the words interdisciplinary, multidisciplinary, transdisciplinary, intradisciplinary, inter-professional, etc., in reference to the topic. We have no doubt inadvertently fallen into the same trap, despite our attempt in the first chapter to define the boundaries of the subject in great detail.

A third observation was that persons involved in the building of teams freely borrowed ideas from the various social sciences and professions to improve the function of teams. Needless to say, while some of these theories concerning organizational, group, and individual behavior are almost directly applicable to teams, others miss the mark. For example, there seem to be many points of incongruence between research findings in small group dynamics and the apparent realities of team dynamics. To examine this aspect, we have initiated some research aimed directly at team situations and have posited the need for a number of studies that would go beyond our current research efforts.

We have attempted to be descriptive and analytical. In those instances where we are prescriptive, we have endeavored either to back such prescriptions with empirical data or indicate to the reader that the statement reflects our particular bias.

In the last few years a number of colleagues have offered support and encouragement for this project. We particularly would like to thank Dean Anne Pascasio and Dr. Molly Vogt of the School of Health Related Professions and Dean James Kelly, Dr. Ralph Peabody, and Dr. Mary Moore of the School of Education of the University of Pittsburgh. In addition, our sincere thanks to Mrs. Irene Petrovich, who typed this manuscript.

We are also very grateful to the many agencies and institutions that have allowed us to study their teams.

Finally, we are particularly grateful to our students for their enthusiasm and interest in this project and for their many helpful comments.

Alex J. Ducanis
and
Anne K. Golin
December 1979

Chapter 1

The Team Approach

More and more in recent years, responsibility for the provision of human services to patients, clients, and others is shared by an interdisciplinary team of professionals. Underlying this development is the major assumption that an interdisciplinary team will bring together diverse skills and expertise to provide more effective, better coordinated, better quality services for clients. On the basis of this belief, the team approach has been adopted in a variety of health and human service settings throughout the country. Yet the implications of the team concept have not always been fully understood, and in some cases early enthusiasm has been followed by disillusionment as the difficulties inherent in the team approach became apparent.

Although the team approach has been widely heralded as a promising innovation in the delivery of human services, to date the concept has generated more rhetoric than research and an adequate theory of teams has yet to be formulated. Before an appropriate conceptual base can be fully developed, there is a clear need for additional research on the use and effectiveness of the human service team. A clearer understanding of the concept could only improve the effectiveness of the team delivery approach.

The present volume brings together the work of several disciplines in an effort to formulate such a conceptual base. Research findings and theoretical concepts from psychology, sociology, management, and decision sciences are integrated and applied to the team process. Existing research is supplemented by studies directed specifically at team functioning. Areas where further research is needed are identified and discussed. Throughout the book there is an attempt to help the professional become aware of the factors that have an impact upon team functions.

In this chapter we examine what is meant by the team approach, see how the concept has developed, describe the characteristics of teams and the variables that affect team functioning, and finally, provide an overview of the material covered in subsequent chapters.

DEFINITIONS OF THE TEAM APPROACH

According to Webster's *Third New International Dictionary* (1976), a *team* may be defined as: "a number of persons associated together in work or activity as: a group of specialists or scientists functioning as a collaborative unit (the diagnostic team of psychiatrist, clinician, and social worker in a child guidance clinic)." The same source defines *teamwork* as: "work done by a number of associates with usually each doing a clearly defined portion but all subordinating personal prominence to the efficiency of the whole (teamwork of a football eleven)."

Collaboration is also the basis of the definition proposed by Rubin, Plovnick, and Fry (1975): "If the basic mission or job required that you and others must work together and coordinate your activities with each other, then you are a team" (p.3).

Parker (1972) points out that the involvement of a number of professionals with a patient does not in itself insure a team approach: "For a team to exist, there must be more than a variety of providers: each provider must function as a sub-unit of a whole in a synergistic relationship" (p. 9). The same point is emphasized again by Wendland and Crawford (1976): "Individuals trained in differing disciplines do not become a team by the mere process of calling themselves one, nor do they manage treatments simply by doing them. What they need is a system set up specifically to effectuate collaboration" (p. 5).

This focus on interprofessional collaboration stems in part from the concept of the "whole person." As Wendland and Crawford (1976) indicate, much of the rationale for the team concept comes from the realization that fragmented care does not really meet the needs of the individual and that

> concern for the patient as a medical, social, psychological, and economic whole in combination with the delivery of ongoing services necessarily requires coordinated efforts. The team must recognize the principle that its specialist members need to become one functioning unit; just as the patient's life is one organismic whole (p.3).

In defining the team concept we find that teams have been variously described as interdisciplinary, multidisciplinary, intradisciplinary, transdisciplinary, intraprofessional, and interprofessional. The use of so many terms and sporadic attempts to draw fine distinctions between them has at times led not to clarification but to even greater confusion. When a team is composed of several members of the same profession (as when two or three dentists are collaborating on the same case), it may appropriately be referred to as an "intraprofessional" team. On the other hand, a dentist, dental hygienist, and dental assistant function together as an intradisciplinary" team. It is more usual to find a team composed of members of a number of different professions, cooperating across disciplines, and in these instances any of the other terms might properly be used. Since in general we are dealing with differences in profession rather than differences in discipline, some may prefer the use of "interprofessional." However, we feel that attempts to distinguish between "interdisciplinary," "multidisciplinary," and "transdisciplinary" team approaches (Hart, 1976; Holm, 1978) may be somewhat premature. At the present time, the study of teams may best be facilitated by the use of a commonly agreed upon term to describe those teams composed of members of different professions. Since "interdisciplinary " is the term most frequently employed in recent literature, it will be used throughout this volume.

In the definitions reviewed above, the essential element seems to be that of collaboration or coordination of services. Therefore, for purposes of this book, *the interdisciplinary team will be defined as a functioning unit, composed of individuals with varied and specialized training, who coordinate their activities to provide services to a client or group of clients.*

DEVELOPMENT OF THE TEAM APPROACH

The team approach is not a recent innovation in health care and human services, although the practice has received increased attention of late. The dangers of specialization and the need for teamwork were discussed in the first quarter of this century by Barker (1922). According to Ackerly, "the psychiatrist, social worker and psychologist were brought together as a full fledged team in the early 20's" (Ackerly, 1947, p. 191). Although the team approach was prominent in child guidance centers long before 1940, the team concept received a major impetus during World War II as reported by Hutt, Menninger, and O'Keefe (1947). Writing in 1953, Drew indicated that the idea of a medical-social work team had already been "worked at" for "more than a quarter of a century." Primary health teams were organized by Martin Cherkasky and later by George Silver in the late 1940s at Montefiore Hospital in the Bronx, spreading to neighborhood health centers under the Office of Economic Opportunity in the 1960s (Kindig, 1975). In 1951 teamwork had become a "fashionable term" in rehabilitation (Whitehouse, 1951), and by 1959 Patterson questioned whether the rehabilitation team had become obsolete (Patterson, 1959).

Over the years the team concept has been applied to child abuse (Martin, 1976; Schmitt, 1978), corrections (Thomas, 1964), exceptional children (Allen, Holm, & Schiefelbusch, 1978; Beck, 1962; Challela, 1979; Hart, 1976; and Sells & West, 1976), chronic illness (Halstead, 1976), long-term care (Melia, 1978), anesthesia (Brown, 1977), community mental health (Lieb, Lipsitch, & Slaby, 1973; Sifneos, 1969; Stueks, 1965), dentistry (Craig, 1970), family health care (Aradine & Hansen, 1970; Bates, Lieberman, & Powell, 1970; Lashof, 1968), as well as to other specific problems. The team approach has also continued to be a major aspect of rehabilitation services (Crisler & Settles, 1979; Jacques, 1970; Wagner, 1977; Wile, 1970; Wilson, 1962).

Although a number of forces were influential in the emergence of the team approach, three major factors seem to have been particularly significant: (1) the concept of the "whole" client, (2) the needs of the organization, and (3) mandates from outside the organizations. Let us briefly examine these factors.

The Concept of the Whole Client

Whitehouse addressed this issue in 1951 when he identified three assumptions in teamwork:

1. The human organism is dynamic and is an interacting, integrated whole.
2. Treatment must be dynamic and fluid to keep pace with the changing person and must consider all that person's needs.
3. Teamwork, an interacting partnership of professionals specializing in these needs and dealing with the person as a whole, is a valid method for meeting these requirements (Whitehouse, 1951, pp. 45-46).

The "whole client" may be a phrase that has become trite through overuse, but the underlying concept remains viable. It reflects the idea that the problems presented by the client are interrelated and cannot be adequately treated in isolation. For example, if a client is being treated for a medical disorder, such as diabetes, without some attention given to how other aspects of the client's life relate to the medical problem, treatment may not be optimally successful. In the case of the diabetes patient, the degree of psychological stress in the job situation and the impact of the client's medical problems on the family are two of the more obvious aspects that need to be examined. Even when a number of problem areas are addressed, the various services provided may be fragmented and uncoordinated, resulting in confusion and apprehension on the part of the client. The team approach has been developed in response to that kind of fragmentation.

The Needs of the Organization

With greater professional specialization has come a significant increase in the number and variety of professionals and paraprofessionals operating within health care and other human service organizations. As more and more individuals become involved in providing services to a particular client, the need for clarifying the lines of communication and authority within the agency becomes increasingly acute. Otherwise the organization, like the client, may suffer from the negative effects of fragmentation. The interdisciplinary team offers a way of organizing personnel to facilitate communication and the exchange of pertinent information concerning the client.

External Mandates

Not only does the organization react to internal rules, it is also responsive to pressures and regulations from without. In recent years the team approach has received considerable impetus from legislative mandates, state and federal government regulations, and the requirements of various third party payers. Team responsibility in assessment, diagnosis, and treatment was seen as one way to improve the quality of care and provide for professional accountability. As a result, a number of health care and related organizations moved to a team system because it was imposed from without, rather than because of any real commitment to such an approach. Unfortunately, teams initiated *solely* because of external mandates sometimes function as teams in name only, with participants simply going through the motions rather than working toward a true coordination of services.

CHARACTERISTICS OF THE TEAM

To further clarify the concept of a team approach we would like to suggest a number of general characteristics common to interdisciplinary teams. It is likely that others may disagree with some of the specific attributes which we have identified, and it may be some time before a firm consensus can be reached concerning those characteristics which are indeed common to all teams. In the meantime, this tentative set of criteria may be useful in deciding whether a specific group should be considered an interdisciplinary team.

Nine characteristics can be identified, and these may be further divided into three main categories: composition, functions, and task.

Composition

1. *A team consists of two or more individuals.* One person does not constitute a team; the nature of teamwork requires the action of two or more persons. Teams can operate as pairs (such as physician and nurse) or as triads (such as psychiatrist, psychologist, and social worker). The two-member team has many of the same needs and characteristics found in larger configurations.

Most members of the interdisciplinary team are usually professionals, but nonprofessionals and paraprofessionals may also be team members. Indeed, the client himself along with members of the client's family may be regarded as part of the team. However, at least *one* team member must be a professional if the group is to be considered a team.

2. *There may be face-to-face or non-face-to-face configurations.* A team may meet regularly with direct and immediate communication. However, the team concept does not necessarily exclude groups that rarely or never meet.

There are instances where communication takes the form of an exchange of written reports or materials. The team may even communicate primarily by telephone or by radio, as used by emergency squads.

3. *There is an identifiable leader.* The leadership of the team may shift due to the changing nature of the task; however, at any point in time the leadership can be identified. Leaderless groups are not teams. Some advocates of the team approach seem to suggest that teams are by definition democratic groups and are neither hierarchial or authoritarian. This seems to be an unduly restrictive view that would rule out groups such as operating room teams, long regarded as classic examples of teamwork. Thus we do not specify the *form* that leadership might take, only that a leader is identifiable.

Functions

Teams can also be characterized by their functions or methods of operation.

4. *Teams function both within and between organizational settings.* The most common type of team is one in which there is a parent organization that provides the support system for the team's operation. Thus we may find teams functioning in schools, rehabilitation centers, and other organizations. However, teams also operate *between* organizations, with professionals from a number of agencies working together on a particular problem or a specific case. For example, the mental health team for a patient living in the community might include representatives from the psychiatric hospital of which the patient is a former resident, the community living facility in which the patient now resides, a counselor from the local community mental health center, and a vocational placement specialist from the vocational training center in which the patient is presently enrolled.

5. *Roles of participants are defined.* Roles of team participants are generally defined in terms of the particular professional competencies of each team member and the nature of the task to be done. Although teams differ in the extent to which roles overlap and conflict, in the clarity of the role definitions, and in the flexibility of established roles, role definition and differentiation is a team characteristic. A group in which each person can and does fill all roles is not a team.

6. *Teams collaborate.* The team is a collaborative endeavor whereby the diverse skills and expertise of team members are combined to provide solutions to specific problems. There seems to be general agreement in the team literature that such coordination of services is a definitive characteristic of teams.

7. *There are specific protocols of operation.* Each team develops certain rules of operation, certain ways of proceeding to accomplish its task. These may range from unwritten group norms of behavior to formal written procedural manuals. In either case, the protocol of operations is empirically identifiable.

Task

In addition, there are certain characteristics associated with the unique task of an interdisciplinary human service or health care team.

8. *The team is client-centered.* The client is the focus of the team's efforts and the reason for the team's existence. While at times it may appear that the team has been formed for the comfort and convenience of its members or the organization, the prime concern of the team is the client.

9. *The team is task oriented.* The team is primarily a task-oriented group that exists to improve the conditions of the client's life by dealing with the problems that have brought the client to the attention of the team.

Again, these nine characteristics are suggested as tentative criteria to be considered in identifying a team. Other attributes could also be included — for example, the team's stability over time. Does the length of time a group is in operation have anything to do with team development? May a group of individuals skilled in teamwork and skilled in their own roles function as a team without going through the various stages of team development identified in the literature?

Another potential characteristic concerns the channels of team communication. Unfortunately, there is not yet sufficient empirical evidence concerning formal and informal communication networks to make this aspect crucial to the identification of a team.

A number of other variables which may prove to be important characteristics common to all teams will be examined in later chapters.

THE TEAM SYSTEM AND THE PLAN OF THIS BOOK

Any attempt to analyze the functioning of an interdisciplinary team quickly points up the need for a theoretical framework that allows us to focus on some of the major dimensions of the team concept and to systematically organize what might otherwise be considered a motley collection of isolated facts about team behavior. While much has been written about the team approach, an adequate theory of interdisciplinary teams in human service institutions has yet to be developed. While it may be premature to formulate a "theory" of interdisciplinary teamwork until more research is conducted, a tentative outline of such a conceptual base may actually stimulate future research and theorizing. The purpose of this section is to suggest some of the major dimensions to explore as we move toward a theory of interdisciplinary teams.

The operation of an interdisciplinary team is the result of a complex interaction of variables associated with the team members, the client, and the context in which the team functions. Figure 1-1 is a schematic representation of the team system and its components. The professionals involved in the team, the client, and the

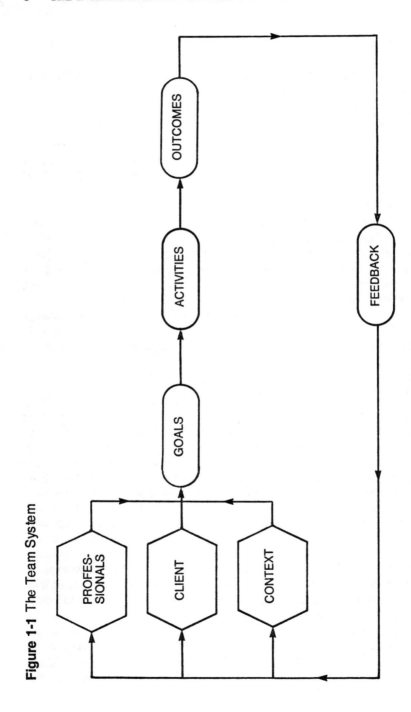

Figure 1-1 The Team System

organizational setting all have an impact on the goals of the team, its activities, and its outcomes. Feedback (formal and informal) provides information concerning outcomes to participants, with resulting changes in goals and activities. The team system serves as the core around which this book is organized.

Professionals

The team is composed of a number of professionals of different theoretical viewpoints, training, and experiences, who differ not only in the resources they bring to the group, but also in role expectations, status, and the extent of their legal responsibility for the client. Among the professions often represented on the team are medicine, nursing, social work, psychology, education, physical and occupational therapy, counseling, and various specialities within these disciplines. Each team is a unique blend of the professional and personal characteristics of its members, its effectiveness determined in large part by the dynamics of that configuration. The similarities, differences, and areas of overlap among the various professions provide a source of potential conflict and misunderstanding that can have considerable impact on team functioning. Chapters Two and Three focus on the professionals involved in the team approach and the relationships among them.

Client

The focus of the services provided by the interdisciplinary team is a patient or client who seeks help for a medical, psychological, educational, or social problem or set of problems. The client may be a passive object of the team's efforts, her or his input limited to providing information to the team. Or the client may be an active member of the team and a participant in the decision-making process. In any case, the client is a crucial component of the team system, and ultimately it is he or she who benefits from the team's effectiveness or suffers from a lack of effectiveness. Chapter Four is devoted to an examination of the client's role in the team system.

Context

Context refers to the organizational setting in which the team operates, the network of services of which it is a part, and the social system in which it is located. Hospitals, rehabilitation centers, schools, and other agencies provide particular organizational structures that markedly affect the operation of the team. The size and type of organization, its referral and treatment policies, its communication channels and administrative structure are some of the variables that comprise the organizational context and are important for a full understanding of the team. These factors are reviewed in Chapter Five.

Goals

Goals are objects or aims that give direction to the team. In order to operate effectively, there must be team agreement on direction. In practice, however, each professional member of the team may have a particular conception of the team goals; the organization in which the team functions may have formally specified particular goals for the team; and the client, too, has in mind certain goals to be met by the team. Thus the team goals may be quite diverse or contradictory. Furthermore, unless the team members perceive some congruence between their own goals and the goals of the team, they may quickly lose interest in participating in the team, with a consequent decrease in team effectiveness. If there is not some minimal sense of shared direction, the team is likely to quite literally fall apart.

Activities

Activities refer to what the team does and how it goes about doing it. Activities include the task-related actions of team participants — diagnostic and treatment activities, decision making, conducting case conferences, and writing reports. The specific nature of these activities is determined by the professionals involved, the problems presented by the clients, the organizational context in which the activities are carried out, and the goals of the team. In addition, the team engages in a number of activities designed to improve or maintain the functioning of the group, including the development of a system of norms, the establishment of communication networks, and other forms of interaction. The goals and activities of the team are explored in Chapters Six and Seven.

Outcomes

Outcomes are those events that occur as a result of the team's activities. A client may recover or die, may undergo successful surgery, may learn appropriate activities of daily living, or experience any one of several alternative outcomes. Ultimately outcomes are a measure of the team's effectiveness, but they also provide feedback that may lead to modification of the team's activities. While many of the outcomes are related to the client, there are also other outcomes related to the participants or to the organization. Chapter Eight deals with evaluating the effectiveness of the team and the measurement of outcomes.

The final two chapters address the future of the interdisciplinary team. In Chapter Nine we discuss how to prepare professionals to be part of a team approach and examine some of the problems of team education. Chapter Ten seeks to integrate and summarize the material of the previous chapters by examining some barriers to teamwork and by exploring some ways to improve team performance.

Chapter 2

The Professions

The professionals who constitute health care and human service teams possess special skills and knowledge that, in part, define their role on the team. However, the term "professional" generally implies more than occupational competence. A number of factors interact to create a unique professional identity.

Paradoxically, professionalization in the human service professions has both facilitated and impeded the development and operation of the interdisciplinary team. The rapid expansion of knowledge in health care and the behavioral sciences, and greater availability of different modalities of treatment, has been accompanied by a dramatic increase in specialization and even subspecialization. These changes have led to a division of labor wherein the physician and other human service professionals have delegated certain aspects of care to other workers, who have themselves then aspired to, and in some cases attained, the title of "professional." These new professionals have in turn delegated some of their duties to other subprofessional workers. Of course, in such a system there is a good chance that the client may receive services that are fragmented and uncoordinated. Recognition of this possibility is one of the reasons behind the development of the team approach. At the same time, there are aspects of professional status and of the professions themselves that may mitigate against the optimal functioning of the interdisciplinary team.

In this chapter we will explore those characteristics of the professions that seem to have an impact upon team function — namely, the nature of a profession, the way in which professions have developed, the manner in which an individual is inducted into a profession, and the relationship between the team approach and the professionalization process.

THE NATURE OF A PROFESSION

Originally, "profession" referred to the act of professing, and according to Hughes (1965), "professionals *profess*. They profess to know better than others the nature of certain matters, and to know better than their clients what ails them or their affairs. This is the essence of the professional idea and the professional claim. From it flow many consequences'' (p. 2).

While many would agree with Hughes that knowledge is one of the attributes characteristic of a profession, there is a surprising lack of consensus about what constitutes a profession. For example, Cogan (1953), following a comprehensive review of the definitions of profession, concludes that "no broad acceptance of any authoritative definition has been observed" (p. 47).

One of the earliest attempts to define a profession was that of Abraham Flexner (1915), whose classic paper is still cited and whose ideas have reappeared in many of the later definitions. Flexner proposed six criteria characterizing a profession: *intellectual activities,* based on *science and learning,* used for *practical purposes,* which can be *taught,* and is *organized internally,* and is *altruistic.* The professions were seen by Flexner as morally superior to other occupations, and he notes that "what matters most is professional spirit. . . . [Since when] accepted professions are prosecuted at a mercenary or selfish level, law and medicine are ethically no better than trades" (p. 590).

It is this sense of altruism or "professional spirit" that has traditionally set the professions not only apart from, but also above other methods of earning a living. Professional work is seen as an end in itself, not merely a means to an end (Greenwood, 1957). Such lofty status serves as a significant incentive for those individuals who hope to become members of the professions and for those occupational groups that are striving toward professionalization.

Much of the confusion and ambiguity associated with "profession" arise from the popular usages of the term. For example, "professional" is sometimes distinguished from "amateur" on the basis of receiving payment for services. It is in this sense that a tennis player, a singer, and a plumber might all be called "professional" even though these occupations differ greatly from the original professional groups (medicine, law, and the clergy).

The difficulties inherent in reaching consensus on the definition of a term that is both a social science concept and a popular expression has led Becker (1962) to take a "radically sociological" viewpoint,

> regarding professions simply as those occupations which have been fortunate enough in the politics of today's work world to gain and maintain possession of that honorific title. On this view, there is no such thing as the "true" profession and no set of characteristics necessarily associated with the title. There are only those work groups which are commonly regarded as professions and those which are not (p. 33).

In contrast to a functional viewpoint of the professions, Bucher and Strauss (1961) outline what they call a *process* approach:

> Functionalism sees a profession largely as a relatively homogeneous community whose members share identity, values, definitions of role, and interests. . . . In actuality, the assumption of relative homogeneity within the professions may not be entirely useful; there are many identities, many values, and many interests (pp. 325-326).

They propose rather, that a profession can be viewed as a "loose amalgamation of segments which are in movement" (p. 333), and they examine the diversities, cleavages, and emerging specializations within the field of medicine.

Sussman (1966) proposes that "the core characteristics of a profession are: *service orientation* and a *body of theoretical knowledge,* with *autonomy of the work group* as a by-product of the two" (p. 184). By service orientation, Sussman refers not only to the notion of altruistic motivation rather than self-interest, but also to the idea that "the community defines the need for the service and accords it varying prestige, status, and power" (p. 184). The second characteristic, a theoretical body of knowledge, refers to abstract information usually acquired during a long period of training. Because of the professional's specialized knowledge and service orientation, the community generally sanctions a greater degree of autonomy for the professional than for members of other occupations. Since professionals possess unique knowledge and skills, they alone are considered capable of judging what is best for the client. As Greenwood (1957) puts it, "the client's subordination to professional authority invests the professional with a monopoly of judgment. When an occupation strives toward professionalization, one of its aspirations is to acquire this monopoly" (p. 48). This greater degree of freedom or autonomy usually necessitates a code of ethics regulating the behavior of members of the profession. However, several recent trends, including the rise of "consumerism," a more knowledgeable public, and increasing governmental intervention seem to be eroding some of the autonomy of the professions.

In addition to these core characteristics, there are a number of other traits associated with professionalism (Goode, 1960; Sussman, 1966). For example, through various professional associations and organizations, a profession is generally able to set standards of ethics and training, and establish criteria for admission to the profession. The profession also "engages in organizational and legislative activities leading to certification and licensure, the legitimization of power and the perpetuation of autonomy" (Sussman, 1966, p. 184).

Although a profession may be identified in this fashion, a number of writers (Goode, 1960; Greenwood, 1957; Sussman, 1966) have pointed out that it may be more reasonable to regard professionalization as a continuum rather than as an all-or-none phenomenon. In this view, an occupation may be regarded as *more* or *less* professional depending on how closely it meets certain adopted criteria. It is to be expected then, that any particular field of service will be staffed by a diversity of occupational groups of varying degrees of professionalization, and that the development and movement of such groups will have major impact on the delivery of services and on the human service team.

THE DEVELOPMENT OF A PROFESSION

Professionalization, and the increased prestige and status associated with it, is the goal of the members of many occupational groups. This is true of those occupations loosely referred to as the health or human service professions. In moving from a nonprofessional or paraprofessional status to that of a "true" profession, these occupations pass through several more or less distinct stages of professionalization, as illustrated in Table 2-1. Along the way, changes can be seen in the social context, in the role definition, and in the knowledge base of the emerging profession. The process begins with the recognition of an unmet social need in Stage I and culminates in Stage IV in external recognition of the autonomy of the profession, the development of a system of professional norms and values, and a growing body of knowledge leading to further specialization within the profession.

As the knowledge base of any profession grows, there is a tendency for individuals to specialize in a particular area. The speciality then goes through a developmental process similar to that of the parent profession, until the new profession gains recognition within the parent profession as well as from the outside community. This process has been illustrated in the health professions whenever physicians have attempted to use others to extend the services provided to patients. Some of these paraprofessional groups have moved through the various stages of professionalization and are now claiming full professional status in their own right. These new professions have in turn spawned additional paraprofessionals. For example, Respiratory Therapists were earlier referred to as Inhalation Therapy Technicians. Now there is a new occupation, Respiratory Therapy Technician, which serves as an aide to the Respiratory Therapist. There are a number of other fields in which individuals who once acted as aides to the physician have in turn developed their own system of aides. An unfortunate side effect of this is that in some professions a rather rigid hierarchical system has been instituted, precluding the development of any rational career ladder.

An important aspect of professionalization is the basic assumption that those who are "higher" in the system possess all of the knowledge and skills of those lower in the hierarchy. When this assumption can no longer be defended, the subordinate group begins the move toward professionalization. Such situations are often fraught with acrimony and rancor and may lead to inter- and intraprofessional strife and rivalry. Typically, each profession becomes more protective of its domain and of its portion of the knowledge base. This occurs both horizontally and vertically. Horizontally, the need for specialization caused by an increase in the knowledge base creates a split between two or more groups of equal status, such as radiologists and anesthesiologists. Vertically, differentiation occurs when one group delegates duties to another group, based upon the aforementioned assumption that the first group is master of the complete knowledge base of the second group. Eventually those considered lower in the hierarchy begin to assert that their knowledge base is indeed specialized and that the higher group is not privy to it.

The medical profession in particular sometimes has difficulty maintaining control of what were vertically subordinate professional groups. As the parent

Table 2-1 Stages of Professionalization

Stage	Social Context	Role Definition	Knowledge Base
I.	Social demand or need to be filled.	Undifferentiated attempts to fill need. Anyone may try (and does).	No unique body of knowledge.
II.	Recognition by society that some fill this need better than others.	Differentiation — some people or group fill need.	Development of a body of knowledge unique to filling needs.
III.	Outside recognition of special group.	Self-recognition and development of means of recognition of who is in group and who is not.	Development of means of induction into group, transmission of knowledge, values, and skills.
IV.	Outside recognition of the right to control group membership.	Regulation of group membership.	Increasing knowledge leading to specialization within role.

profession for a number of other groups, physicians see themselves as having the ultimate moral, legal, and ethical responsibility for the welfare of the client, but see their authority being diffused and eroded as their knowledge base is spread among a number of other professions and paraprofessional groups.

As new professions emerge, there is a tendency to delegate the more routine tasks to lower levels of workers. Thus the human service occupations take the form of a pyramid that grows from the bottom and at the same time widens its base. Figure 2-1 shows this hierarchical pyramid with some illustrative occupational groups.

Since the physician is given ultimate responsibility for the client in matters of health care (and thus is located at the top of the pyramid), it might appear that as the pyramid grows in size with more and more occupational groups included, the power of the physician would increase concomitantly. In actuality, the physician

Figure 2-1 Hierarchical Relationships in the Professions

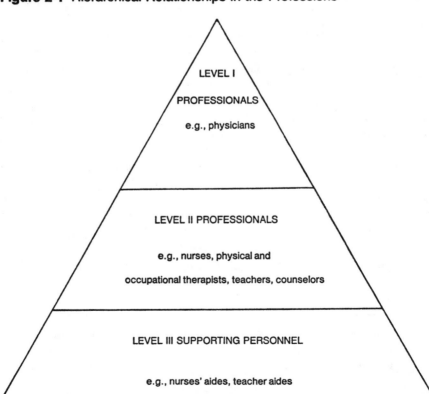

LEVEL I

PROFESSIONALS

e.g., physicians

LEVEL II PROFESSIONALS

e.g., nurses, physical and

occupational therapists, teachers, counselors

LEVEL III SUPPORTING PERSONNEL

e.g., nurses' aides, teacher aides

becomes more dependent on a larger number of workers to carry out his or her orders. As the treatment group enlarges, there are more problems in communication, in lines of authority, and in areas of responsibility. As the treatment process becomes more complex, the physician cannot personally oversee every step in the client's treatment and so delegates more and more responsibilities to others and depends on them to fulfill these obligations.

Coordination becomes a serious problem as the size of the group increases. The team approach is one way to provide coordination, and the physician may be willing to delegate some responsibility for treatment and decision making to the team itself. This is likely to occur when the physician has already experienced some loss of control over the treatment process because of the number of workers involved in the case and the difficulty in directly supervising all of them. In this kind of situation the team approach is one way to provide that supervision.

A CASE STUDY OF PROFESSIONALIZATION

The process by which an occupational group evolves into a profession may be illustrated by a brief review of the development of physical therapy. One of several newly emerging health professions to appear in this century, the history of physical therapy has been recorded by a number of authors (Beard, 1961; Johnson, 1971; Pascasio, 1966; Vogel, 1967).

While it may be, as Johnson (1971) suggests, that ancient peoples used sunlight, water, and massage as primitive forms of therapy, physical therapy as a profession probably began with World War I when the need to rehabilitate large numbers of young soldiers gave impetus to this form of treatment. The demand for trained personnel in the U.S. Army led to the development of a course of training at Walter Reed Hospital and to a request that colleges with physical education programs assist in the training of "reconstruction aides." By the close of the war some 800 aides were in service, and the need for a physical therapy component of medical care had been established (Vogel, 1967). In January 1921 the American Women's Physical Therapeutic Association was established with some 200 members. The first steps toward professionalization had been taken.

The purpose of the association is described by Beard (1961):

> The objectives set forth in the constitution were: (1) to establish and maintain a professional and scientific standard for those engaged in the profession of physical therapeutics; (2) to increase efficiency among its members by encouraging them in advanced study; (3) to disseminate information by the distribution of medical literature; (4) to make available efficiently trained women to the medical profession; and (5) to sustain social fellowship and intercourse upon grounds of mutual interest (p. 844).

Among the membership requirements was training at a recognized school of physiotherapy. In 1922 the name of the association was changed to the American Physiotherapy Association, and membership was opened to men.

In 1925 the American Medical Association established a Council on Physical Therapy and called for courses in physical therapy in medical schools. At about the same time the American Physiotherapy Association developed curriculum guidelines and set minimum standards for the training of its professionals. The proposed curriculum was a nine-month, 1,200-hour program for graduates of physical education or nursing schools and was published in the *P.T. Review* and the *Journal of the American Medical Association*. In 1930 eleven schools were approved by the association as training sites. In 1934 the American Medical Association was asked to assume responsibility for the review of educational facilities, and in 1936 the AMA Council on Medical Education and Hospitals published the "Essentials of an Acceptable School for Physical Therapy Technicians." These standards were quite similar to the minimum standards developed earlier by the physical therapists.

Pascasio (1966) describes the content of the suggested curriculum:

> Excluding the 400 hours allotted to clinical experience and considering only the didactic portion of the curriculum, basic sciences accounted for 41 percent of the course. Physical therapy procedures totaled 33 percent, while 21 percent was devoted to the study of ethics and physical therapy as applied to various medical specialities. The remaining 5 percent was to be divided among electives, all of which were of a professional nature (p. 5).

An official journal of the association, the *P.T. Review*, had begun in 1921 as a quarterly publication and became bimonthly in 1928 (Beard, 1961). In 1927 the constitution was revised and a new statement appeared: "to cooperate with, or under, the direction of the medical profession and to provide a central registry which will make available to the medical profession efficiently trained assistants in physical therapy" (Beard, 1961, p. 846). This attitude is also reflected in a quotation from an early issue of the association's journal: "We must in this (standards of practice) stick to our own field which is the carrying out of prescriptions given by doctors and not diagnosing, prescribing, or in any way experimenting in the treatment of disease" (Beard, p. 847).

As the profession grew, so did its association, and Beard delineates various steps in this process, from the hiring of a part-time secretary to the employment of an executive director in 1944. The reported membership of the association grew steadily, with 4,104 members in 1950, 8,474 in 1960, and approximately 14,000 by 1970. In the meantime, the number of approved training institutions had increased to 64 in 1970, with 45 of those awarding a baccalaureate degree, 15 a certificate (either post-baccalaureate or concomitant with a bachelor's degree), and 4 offering a master's degree (Johnson, 1971).

In terms of the characteristics described by Sussman (1966), discussed earlier in this chapter, physical therapy clearly demonstrates a strong service orientation and a theoretical body of knowledge. Society recognized the need for its services during two major wars and a serious epidemic of poliomyelitis in 1944.

The question of professional autonomy is a more complex one. The degree of autonomy accorded physical therapy is not clear, particularly in view of its subordinate relationship to the medical profession. Physical therapy has engaged in several of the activities that Sussman has called professional *traits:* development of an association, legislative activities, development of standards of training and admission to the profession, publication of a professional journal and of a code of ethics. The continued emphasis on a strong science component in the education of physical therapists and the recent emergence of advanced programs at the doctoral level support the idea that this speciality has indeed come a long way toward professionalization. In many ways the growth of physical therapy parallels that of many midlevel or Level II professions that have emerged in this century.

INTERNAL CONTROL OF PROFESSIONS

Many of the professions represented on the human service team are presently in a state of flux. Some are moving toward greater professionalization, some seem to be losing prestige and power, and others are plagued by internal dissension and fragmentation as a result of increased specialization within the field. The role expectations and actual behavior of the individual team member will be greatly influenced by the stability or conflict within the profession. Indeed, conflict within the emerging or changing profession can have a marked impact on the operation of the team itself. Therefore we will briefly examine some of the sources of conflict that may affect the team and how this conflict is controlled by the professions.

According to Parsons (1959) there are two main types of professional groups: those formed in the workplace by the employing organization (a school or hospital) and those formed by individuals. Of the two, it is the latter that plays the major role in professionalization and deals with intraprofessional conflict.

> The main thrust toward professionalization by marginal occupations comes through the association organized by leaders of the field. Its major activities are to provide the conditions for all its members to function as professionals, serving the society, increasingly utilizing a growing body of theoretical knowledge and obtaining a payoff in prestige and financial rewards (Sussman, 1966, p. 191).

We have already seen the role played by the association of physical therapists in the professionalization of that occupation. Often the professional association will establish an official journal or some other mechanism for communicating with members, promoting the profession, and exerting control over professional activities.

The attempt to establish a professional identity and draw boundaries between itself and other professions or specialities may serve as an integrative force within the emerging profession. At the same time, there may be a number of factors leading to fragmentation and conflict within the group. As Goode (1960) puts it, "no occupation, then, becomes a profession without a struggle" (p. 902). The external conflict with other professions has often been noted. "If a new occupation claims the right to solve a problem which formerly was solved by another, that claim is an accusation of incompetence and the outraged counteraccusation is, of course, 'encroachment' " (Goode, 1960, p. 902). Goode illustrates this point with the conflict between two emerging professional specialities, clinical psychology and psychiatry, a battle that has continued over a period of several years.

External threats by other professions are not infrequent, but in some cases such *interprofessional* conflict can lead to a pulling together of disparate interests within the threatened group and a submerging of internal differences, at least temporarily. On the other hand, *intraprofessional* conflicts precipitated by professionalization are less obvious and often overlooked, but these may actually be much more disruptive to the emerging profession than external threats.

As long as the professional organization serves primarily to provide mutual support and help in solving the typical problems members face in carrying out their professional duties, then its effect will be primarily an integrative one. However, as the push for professionalization grows stronger, the membership may be far from unanimous in their support of these efforts, and "reactionaries" within the profession may become more vocal in their opposition to the proposed changes.

As the group moves toward further professionalization, the association usually includes among its goals: increasing the length and difficulty of professional preparation, raising standards for admission to training programs, and establishing licensure and/or certification requirements. However, these goals may not be supported by all members of the professional organization. As Sussman (1966) points out, the rank and file may not move as quickly as the leaders of the emerging professions. Furthermore, the move to raise standards may be thought to imply some degree of incompetence among the present ranks, and the establishment of new and more rigid requirements for membership may be seen as a threat by older members. Although "grandfathering" provisions are often included to reduce resistance to change, such arrangements may be seen as leading to a kind of second-class citizenship within the profession. While some attempts may be made to upgrade the less qualified members, Sussman indicates that the price of professionalization may be to award status and prestige to some who are "undeserving" with the hope that they will quickly leave the field.

For many members, the promise of greater economic rewards, prestige, and power serves as a strong incentive, and the majority of the membership may give full support to the association's moves toward professionalization. However, according to Bucher and Strauss (1961), "associations are not everybody's association but represent one segment or a particular alliance of segments" of the profession (p. 33). The various segments within a profession (or even within a speciality within a profession) may differ in terms of perceived mission, work activities, methodology and techniques, relationships with clients, sense of colleagueship, interests, and associations. This diversity may not be apparent to outsiders who respond to the public image projected by the professional association and its leaders. Yet this public image may reflect only the power of particular segments within the organization, rather than represent the unified position of the total membership (Bucher & Strauss, 1961).

For individual team members, the political machinations within the professional association may have little meaning except as they influence professional roles or how others perceive those roles. However, insofar as the conflicts within the profession make roles ambiguous and provide a misleading view of responsibilities, they may interfere with how team members function, both with clients and with other team members. If the profession has not adequately conveyed an appropriate image to outsiders, individual members may find it necessary to spend an inordinate amount of time clarifying their role on the team. It should be noted, however, that a certain amount of role "flexibility" is desirable for effective team functioning; overly rigid definition of professional roles may prohibit "give and take" and fail to provide opportunities for role negotiation that can be important to the smooth functioning of the team. If the professional association is too restrictive in its regulation of the professional activities of its members, professionals may find serious conflicts between their roles as team members and the role expectations of the professional association.

EXTERNAL CONTROL OF PROFESSIONS

While a great deal has been written about the autonomy of the professions and their ability to regulate themselves, there are differences between professions in how much professional autonomy is exercised and who decides how much autonomy is allowed. Close examination reveals there is a great deal of variation in the degree of external control exerted upon the professions.

External controls are exercised in a number of ways, including governmental licensure and regulation. The professional associations attempt to exert control within the profession by certification and disciplinary procedures. However, the associations may also attempt to exert control over the practice of other professions, particularly when one profession sees its prerogatives eroded or usurped by another. Another means of external control is the accreditation of educational programs by external agencies. We noted in our discussion of the professionalization of physical therapy that the process of approval of training programs was taken over by the Council of the American Medical Association. Individual organizations and institutions, hospitals, schools, and clinics maintain control over who may practice or provide services and thus also exert some control over the professions.

Such controls have clear implications for the operation of the human service team, since they have impact on who does what, who is responsible for supervision, and the scope and limits of a particular profession. Interestingly, the impetus for external recognition and control has often come from within the particular professional group, as when the physical therapy association requested that the AMA assume responsibility for the approval of its educational programs.

Some of the factors that may lead a profession to seek governmental regulation through licensure or similar statutes are:

1. an inability to prevent those who are considered unqualified from practicing
2. the need to define and protect the scope of practice on a statutory basis
3. the need for legal status to assure recognition for purposes such as third party payment requirements or federal funding programs for student support.

Each of these factors may influence the way professionals interact in an interdisciplinary team. For example, if unqualified persons are using the title of a particular profession, the integrity of that profession may be questioned by other professionals on the team and members of that profession may lose status within the team. The competence of all practitioners of that profession is called into question since there is no way to judge whether in fact the individual is a professional or a charlatan.

A second important factor is the apparent need to legally define the boundaries of the profession. This has two purposes: to ensure that these areas of professional practice will not be encroached upon by other professions, and to retain exclusive rights to as many professional prerogatives as possible. An example of action on the part of one profession to prevent what was believed to be encroachment, and reaction to it, is found in Goode (1960):

Clinical psychologists are newcomers, and have not been in a position to attack the psychiatrists officially, but the latter (with the support and sometimes under the pressure, of the A.M.A.) as the entrenched group have tried in various ways to prevent any infiltration by the former.

Goode cites a number of instances in which the medical profession has opposed certification and licensure of psychologists and has restricted the role of psychologists in mental hospitals. He notes that:

> In 1957, the A.M.A. Council reaffirmed its earlier position that the application of psychological methods to the treatment of illness is a medical function, although psychologists and others may properly be used by medical men in contributory roles when supervised by a physician (p. 909).

This conflict is summarized by Goode: "While clinical psychologists feel that they are being kept from their rightful domain by an intransigent foe, medical men see themselves inundated and infiltrated" (p. 909).

It is clear that the medical profession at that time saw the distinct possibility of some usurpation of their field and used whatever means were at their disposal to stifle it. Clearly such interprofessional disputes do not help facilitate the functioning of an interdisciplinary team. Even for individual teams that function well on the basis of individual respect and trust, there may be a background of interprofessional strife. Often this strife is not apparent to outsiders, but nevertheless manifests itself in ways that are dysfunctional to team operation.

An example of an attempt to define and retain a professional prerogative is seen in a statement about speech pathologists and audiologists who sought licensure in a particular state:

> An attorney general's opinion concerning an individual who was not a physician and who advertised speech and hearing therapy stated that therapy could be considered a medical sub-speciality and that the person offering therapy probably should be a physician or an individual working under the direct supervision of a physician (Nicolais, 1976, p. 22).

Speech pathologists considered it to be an infringement upon their assumed right to work on a *referral* basis without postreferral supervision by a physician, so they sought legal status to clarify the issue. The question of who may perform or prescribe therapy and under what type of supervision is a critical one for the team. As more and more specialities are developed and the knowledge base grows, it becomes impossible for one person to master all of that knowledge or even any major part of it. In the case of the attorney general's opinion given above, is it possible for *any physician* to monitor the work of a speech pathologist or audiologist or is it necessary for that physician to be a master of that area? As the scope of human services and health care are redefined to include the total individual, it becomes increasingly unlikely that *any one* person will be able to adequately monitor that care.

The third reason for seeking governmental sanction is that of legal recognition as a profession. In a sense this ensures that when legislation is drafted the profession will be taken into account. For example, when government grants or fellowships are made available, it is much more likely that those professional areas already sanctioned will receive a share of such support. This "official" recognition confers a certain status on the profession and lends a certain aura of protection to the client who assumes that some responsible party (in this case the government) is overseeing the operation of that profession.

Another type of external control is exercised through the process of accrediting the institutions that educate persons for the profession. In this instance, certain minimum standards may be imposed on an emerging profession by an already existing superordinate profession. An example of this may be found in the position of the American Medical Association's Council on Medical Education, a position probably best expressed by this statement from their board of trustees:

> Every health occupation owes its existence to the need for some patient service. And where the care of the patient is concerned, the physician has a legal, a moral and an ethical responsibility which he cannot avoid. Allied health workers share the responsibility, but only the physician has responsibility which extends over the complete range of patient services. As the major professional association for practicing physicians, A.M.A. feels keenly its responsibility to all physicians to provide coordination and direction to allied health education, in order that appropriate standards for patient services may be established and maintained. . . . There is great interest today in the development of interdisciplinary educational programs in which the physician and various allied health workers will learn together the health team approach to the care of patients. This would appear to call for increasing cooperation between medicine and allied health disciplines in the *maintainance (sic)* of education standards (*Allied Medical Education Directory*, 1976, p. 59).

The 1976 edition of the *Allied Medical Education Directory* identifies 26 "occupations" accredited by the Council on Medical Education. The Council collaborates with 29 different organizations in the development of educational standards for various health occupations. For example, the Joint Review Committee for Respiratory Therapy Education is sponsored by the American Association for Respiratory Therapy, the American College of Chest Physicians, the American Society of Anesthesiologists, and the American Thoracic Society. Educational programs in Respiratory Therapy are evaluated in light of the standards adopted by the Council on Medical Education and the collaborating organizations. Similar procedures are used in developing and evaluating appropriate educational programs in other allied health occupations.

The collaborating organizations also constitute a Panel of Consultants which in addition includes special advisors who come from governmental agencies (such as Health, Education and Welfare and the Veteran's Administration) as well as from private associations (such as the American Association of State Colleges and Universities). This panel meets with a committee of the AMA to "discuss and decide" other matters regarding allied health education. In any case, the final decision in matters of education standards and accreditation, as well as in "other matters" concerning allied health education, rests with the Council and/or the House of Delegates of the American Medical Association. It is therefore the AMA that is listed by the U.S. Office of Education as the accrediting agency for a majority of the allied health occupations. This means the AMA is in an excellent position to exert strong influence on many of the professions that compose the interdisciplinary team. Not only has the AMA exercised strong leadership in the development of many of the allied health professions, it has also maintained a position that ensures its influence. Thus it is not surprising that physicians expect that allied health professionals on the team will relate to them in a manner consistent with the status relationship between their respective professions, at times regarding the allied health professional as an "aide" or "helper."

BECOMING A PROFESSIONAL

Up to now our discussion has focused on the professions themselves, rather than on the individuals who make up those groups. Now let us look briefly at the socialization process whereby the individual acquires the skills and roles of the profession, and at the same time adopts its norms and values. As Vollmer and Mills (1966) point out, "becoming a professional is a gradual process — it doesn't happen all at once" (p. 87). It is a process that begins long before the candidate is admitted to a professional school and long before a final career choice is made. Attitudes toward specific professions may originate in childhood, shaped by real-life experiences with doctors, teachers, dentists, and so forth, and also by what the child reads, sees, or hears concerning these roles. These early attitudes may be unspoken or even unconscious and are usually modified by later experience and information, but nonetheless the early impressions will have an impact on the eventual career choice.

At the point of admission to a professional school, the student may have a hazy, perhaps even romanticized notion of what the professional role entails. Thus an important function of professional training is to initiate trainees into the "culture" of the profession and to develop in them a more realistic expectation of the role to be played. The student gradually becomes aware of the explicit and implicit norms that govern the behavior of members of the profession and may adopt as role models those professionals whose skills he or she particularly admires.

Professional training is long and expensive. This fact alone has shaped the composition of the professions in the United States. Until recent years, children from families of moderate means were often unable to stay in school long enough to complete professional training. Expensive education was beyond their reach. Despite recent attempts to increase the proportion of low-income and minority students in professional training programs and to provide financial assistance for such students, the older well-established professions have not altered much in composition.

Typically as an occupational group moves toward greater professionalization, there is an increase in the length of training. Usually this involves requiring more prerequisites and more coursework and internship-type experiences. However, unless the profession can offer sufficient gains in status and economic incentives, the training period cannot be unduly lengthened (Hughes, 1965).

Increased selectivity in admissions, like length of training, is another sign of greater professionalization. The better established professions that offer greater prestige and potential economic rewards are likely to attract large numbers of persons wishing to enter their ranks. Thus they can also maintain the highest standards of selectivity. These standards are likely to be upheld not only by the faculty of the training institution, but also by the professional association, since greater selectivity further increases the status of the profession. In those professions of highest prestige, criteria not necessary or relevant to the development of needed skills may be used to screen applicants. Minority groups have long been familiar with the "hidden" criteria that sometimes underlie the admissions process. Often women found admission to medical or law schools difficult because, as they were told, they lacked the "motivation" of men, and would "leave the field" to keep house and raise children.

Professions of lower status have traditionally been unable to maintain the stringent requirements of law and medicine, not because these fields were less crucial to meeting social or individual needs, but because the fewer numbers of applicants in relation to places available did not allow for such selectivity. On the other hand, the shorter periods of training in the less prestigious professions meant less initial expense, and apprentice professionals could more quickly begin to regain a return on their educational investment. Thus professions such as nursing and social work became an avenue of social mobility for students of moderate income, for women, and for minority groups.

In some instances, outside sources play a role in "professionalizing" an occupation by providing training funds or scholarships to attract promising candidates into an area of manpower shortage. The federal government has played a major role in the upgrading of a number of professions by making available to students federal stipends for professional training and providing training monies to the university for faculty support and associated expenses. In this manner, universities were offered incentives to provide training programs in areas that Congress felt to be of high priority, and at the same time students who might not have otherwise considered it were encouraged by the available support to enter professional training. The governmental agency administering the federal grant monies also often provided guidelines for such program components as curricular content and admission standards and also developed the procedures for program review. Eventually, the federal funds were decreased, and the university was expected to take over the bulk of the expense of the program so that federal funds could be moved to other programs designed to meet newly emerging needs.

One of the difficulties faced by professional schools is the collection of data by which to validate admission criteria. Often the university faculty members with major responsibility for admission decisions have neither the time nor the financial resources available to carefully test out the predictions that an admissions decision implies. In effect, the acceptance of an applicant into a professional program involves two predictions:

1. This candidate will successfully complete the training program.
2. The applicant will be a successful practitioner of the profession.

Leaving aside for the moment the ambiguities and methodological difficulties inherent in that term "successful," we can see that the more closely the training program simulates professional practice, the easier it is to predict the successful student will become a successful professional. Of course, it is not unusual to find brilliant and talented students who fail to live up to the promise of their training days when they enter the "real" world. However, it is the difficulty in measuring "success" that poses the greatest problems for faculty admission committees. Too often they seize upon whatever "hard" data happens to be available (such as grade point average or test scores) because they cannot, with the resources available, carefully judge the actual effectiveness of their graduates as professionals.

The socialization process does not necessarily end with the granting of a professional degree. As noted earlier, the more established the profession and the higher its status, the longer the period of apprenticeship. In medicine, for example, internships, residencies, and specialized training extend long past the traditional four years of medical school. The development of a private practice and a referral system and acceptance into a major hospital as a staff member are part of the long-term process of establishing a medical career.

In the Level II professions, such as teaching or social work, the period of preparation may be considerably shorter. However, in these professions, too, receiving a degree and getting a job is only the beginning. As many new professionals can attest, it may take many months or even years of experience before one earns full acceptance as a member of the profession. Teachers, for example, may be awarded only temporary certification until further education and/or experience is acquired. Full acceptance as a professional is based not only on proven skill and expertise in the tools of the profession, but also in many cases depends on how well the initiate carries out role expectations.

We have mentioned that the choice of a professional career is determined in part by attitudes toward that career formed early in life. It should be noted that such a choice also depends on the individual's self-image; the career chosen is likely to be one not markedly inconsistent with the individual's self-concept. Where there is a significant discrepancy between one's view of the professional role and the image of oneself, the socialization process will involve a major alteration in one or both of these perceptions. Even when one feels that the chosen career is a "natural" one for them, the individual's professional education will involve a gradual internalization of "a professional image which becomes a very significant aspect of the self-concept" (Vollmer and Mills, 1966, p. 98). The internalization of new roles and changes in self-image have several implications for professional education:

1. Such changes take time and cannot be unduly rushed.
2. Self-concept depends not only on internal reactions but also on the reactions of others.
3. An opportunity to "practice" the role is necessary.

Changes in self-concept require an arena in which to test out new skills and perceptions and to receive confirmation from others. To a great extent, we feel like a professional when others behave toward us as though we are a professional. This generally happens when the student is placed in a field training situation and is expected to play a professional role. As clients and coworkers begin to respond to the student with acceptance and respect, the student plays the role with increasing confidence and authority. Thus he is encouraged to "try on" the professional role under the watchful eye of a supervisor who is likely to focus not only on the development of specific skills but also on the professional image the student projects. The student learns to *act* like a professional as well as to *be* one.

During the process of socialization, the would-be professional may find that the new role is not always congruent with previous roles, and the trainee may begin to experience role conflict. Expectations of others may be such that they demand mutually exclusive behaviors, and the student is forced to either compromise certain roles or abandon them altogether. Conflicts between private and public responsibilities are obvious and not unusual, as when the busy physician or lawyer compromises his or her role as spouse or parent in order to meet professional obligations.

Equally important, although less obvious, are the conflicts between the various professional roles the individual is expected to fill. For example, the apprentice professional may be expected to demonstrate the responsibility and autonomy of a professional, but at the same time play the role of student in interactions with supervisors and teachers. This inconsistency can lead to confusion and anxiety that may interfere with performance in both roles. Such conflicts are not limited to students; established professionals also experience role conflicts and find themselves forced to establish priorities in their activities in order to resolve real or potential conflicts in expectations. In a later chapter we will examine the conflicts between one's professional role and role as a team member — conflicts that seem to be inherent in the team approach.

Some conflicts seem inherent in the nature of the profession itself, and a great deal of time and effort may be spent in attempts to clarify role expectations for the profession as a whole. The conflict of the "scientist-professional" model in clinical psychology has absorbed that profession for over twenty years without clear resolution. Clinical training programs, internship facilities, professional organizations, and individual psychologists have all felt the impact of the conflict between the roles of scientist-researcher and professional practitioner. University professors often experience similar conflicts with regard to expectations stemming from their roles in teaching, scholarly activity, and public service. Since the reward system for professional activities, in terms of status and money, is presumably tied to effective performance in expected roles, the conflict can be a very real one for the individual. Because establishing oneself in a professional career is a long-range endeavor, the young professional is often forced to make decisions regarding role priorities rather early in his or her career, although the results of those decisions may not become clear for some time.

Among the roles in which the professional is expected to engage are those involving interaction with members of other professional groups. One aspect of the role of the psychiatric social worker, for example, is to work with the psychiatrist in implementing treatment plans. The special education teacher must often coordinate her activities with the school psychologist and the regular classroom teacher. Many of the roles of nursing personnel revolve around their interaction with physicians. Human service professionals in general must learn what to expect of other members of the team, and to fill one's role appropriately and effectively one must be sensitive to differences in status and power associated with various role positions.

PROFESSIONAL STATUS

One of the factors that affects the way in which professionals interact on the team is status. It is important here to differentiate between *individual status* which may be conferred upon a team member for various reasons related to her or his performance on the team, and *professional status* which is accorded an individual because of her or his professional identification. Before we look briefly at the concept of status and the relative status positions of some of the human service professions represented on the interdisciplinary team, it should be noted that most studies of professional status have used populations of lay persons to rate the relative status of various occupational groups. In some instances there have been interprofessional comparisons, with various professions ranking each other's relative importance; however, for the most part studies have resorted to the general population for such rankings. To what extent these lay attitudes are representative of attitudes *between* professions is not clear.

Treiman (1977) in a major review of investigations of professional status, yields some interesting results concerning the health professions by comparing rankings across nations. Eighty-five occupational prestige studies conducted in 60 different countries were located and evaluated. These studies were then analyzed and a "prestige score" was computed for each of the occupational categories. From data presented in the appendix of the study, it is possible to examine results for several of those professions found on an interdisciplinary team. It is clear from the data that the physician has a distinct edge in prestige over all others in the health field, with the dentist second.

The human service professions tend to be at the high end of the scale as compared with others. However, such status in relation to other occupations means little *within* the human service system, since the main consideration here is to determine status *among* the particular professions involved in the team. Thus we see a group of rather highly regarded persons who have gained the sanction of society as a whole, yet may still be encumbered by a system that gives more status and privilege to one profession than to another. What is important in the study of team processes is how the various members of the team view each other. These perceptions are the subject of the next chapter.

Chapter 3

Interprofessional Relationships

An essential aspect of the interdisciplinary team is the ability of two or more professionals to work together; this is true whether they are of the same or differing professions. However, the potential misperceptions and misunderstandings are usually greater *between* than *within* professions because the professional is often not really aware of the specific competencies and roles of members of different professions. Overlapping roles, status differences, and differences in viewpoint can easily lead to interprofessional conflict and thus create discord within the team.

Relationships among team members is an important determinant of team effectiveness. Conflict and misperceptions among professionals can seriously interfere with collaborative efforts (Banta and Fox, 1972; Jacobson, 1974). As Frank (1961) points out, professional education involves learning the language, assumptions, and conceptual framework of a particular profession. While this training enhances intraprofessional communication, it may create barriers between professionals in an interdisciplinary team.

> "Obviously if each person in a team of interdisciplinary or interprofessional practitioners relies upon the concepts and assumptions of his discipline or profession and expresses these in whatever he says and does, his attempts at communication to the others will be likely to fail, especially if he is not wholly aware of his own preconceptions and ignores those of his colleagues" (Frank, 1961, p. 1,801).

Professional *ethnocentrism,* differences in professional *status,* and a *lack of understanding* of other professions were cited as primary barriers to communication between professionals by Haselkorn (1958). *Fear of encroachment* by other professionals and *language barriers* can also impede interprofessional collaboration. How well the team handles such barriers may determine its ultimate effectiveness.

INTERPROFESSIONAL PERCEPTIONS

Rubin and Beckhard (1972) in discussing the factors that influence the effectiveness of health teams indicate the importance of expectations about the behavior of other team members. "Each person, in effect, has a set of expectations of how each of the other members should behave as the group works to achieve its goals" (p. 319). These expectations may lead to role ambiguity, role conflict, or role overload for team members.

Horwitz (1969) elaborates on the perceptions of each team member and suggests that there may be considerable discrepancy among the different viewpoints. According to Horwitz, the professional develops four images in his interaction with the team:

1. a personal and professional self-image,
2. expectations of his own profession in that setting,
3. an understanding of the skills and responsibilities of his colleagues, and
4. a perception of his colleagues' image of him.

Using social workers as an example, Horwitz indicates that their self-perception includes how they see themselves helping clients and the kind of social worker they envision themselves to be. Their expectations of social work in the particular setting in which they are working include those activities which they see as "proper" for a social worker under those conditions. Their image of their colleagues is based upon the colleagues' professional skills and responsibilities and personality characteristics. Their opinions regarding their colleagues' image of them include the belief that colleagues see them as a "skillful co-worker," as "likeable but unneeded," or as a "walking encyclopedia."

As Horwitz sums up:

> These images to which the social worker (consciously or unconsciously) refers as he practices are paralleled, of course, in the minds of each of his colleagues. And we bear in mind as we scrutinize the crosscurrents of team practice that the vision people have of their world materially affects the way they conduct themselves within it. Each worker on the team . . . tries to adapt his overtures toward colleagues to the picture of each he has developed in his own mind. Yet each of the others may think of himself as quite different from the portraits the social worker has painted (1969, p. 38).

In an attempt to examine perceptions of one's own professional role and the roles of other team members, Banta and Fox (1972) conducted a series of interviews with physicians, nurses, and social workers who had participated in a health team project in a poverty area. Subjects were asked to describe their own professional colleagues as well as members of the two other professional groups. This method led to the identification of a number of specific interprofessional role strains in the teams. In regard to the sources of strain between the public health nurses and the social workers, the authors note that "These two groups, involved in similar tasks, differed strikingly in social background, in the processes of professional socialization they had undergone, and, to a significant degree, in their professional ethos" (Banta and Fox, 1972, p. 718).

In a discussion of the changing roles of nurses and the need for nurses to work collaboratively with other professions, Stueks (1965) identifies four significant elements in collaboration: *professional identity, professional integrity, overlapping of roles,* and *flexibility.* To avoid role ambiguity and stereotypes, the nurse needs to communicate with other professionals regarding roles and professional identity. Furthermore,

> "if the nurse's professional role is confusing to others, then the roles of other professionals may be equally unclear to the nurses. The nurse may have stereotypes of other professionals, or may not understand them simply because of a lack of contact and experience with them" (Stueks, 1965, p. 317).

Thus we see that members of the team come together with certain preconceptions about their own roles and the roles of other professionals on the team. Perceptions may differ considerably from one professional group to another, and the way that members of a profession such as medicine perceive themselves may be very different from the way doctors are seen by other professionals such as nurses or social workers. Although some degree of difference is unavoidable, extreme perceptual dissonance among team members can be disruptive to efforts at coordination.

The Interprofessional Perception Scale

To examine how professionals view themselves, view other professions, and think other professions view them, a scale of interprofessional perception was developed by the authors (Ducanis and Golin, 1978). The Interprofessional Perception Scale (IPS) is based upon the interpersonal perception method developed earlier by Laing, Phillipson, and Lee (1966) to study several levels of perspective operating in a dyadic relationship, such as that between husband and wife. Alperson (1975) analyzed Laing's method by means of Boolean algebra in order to clarify the underlying truth-functional structures of the method. Alperson concluded that the approach is adaptable to a variety of investigations, including group perceptions.

Basically, Laing's formulation asserts that there are several levels of perspective which each member of a dyadic relationship has of one another. He terms these:

1. *perspective*, i.e., what I say
2. *meta-perspective*, i.e., how I say you would answer the same question
3. *meta-meta-perspective*, i.e., what I say you would say that I said.

To use one of Laing's items as an example, a husband, given the statement "I love her," is asked to answer in three ways:

1. perspective — either "yes" or "no"
2. meta-perspective — how does he think his wife will respond to the statement "he loves me"?
3. meta-meta-perspective — how does he think his wife would say *he* responded?

The Interprofessional Perception Scale also involves three levels of response as it asks a professional to give an opinion of another profession (Level I), tell how members of that profession would respond (Level II), and finally, tell how those professionals would say he or she responded (Level III). Thus, the IPS yields data regarding how a professional views another profession, whether he or she thinks that members of that profession agree or disagree with that view, and whether they understand that perception. The scale can also be used to indicate how subjects see their *own* profession and whether they think other professionals agree with or understand this perception.

Figure 3-1 Sample Response to IPS Item

Item	Level I How would you answer?		Level II How would they answer?		Level III How would they say you answered?	
	True	False	True	False	True	False
The relations between nurses and physicians are very good.	[ ]	[x]	[x]	[ ]	[x]	[ ]

As you can see, this approach can become quite complex. Therefore an example from an early version of the IPS may be helpful to the reader. (See Figure 3-1). The respondent in this example is a nurse. The respondent is asked to answer in three ways: how she would answer, how a physician would answer, and how the physician would say she answered. In this case she responds *false* to the statement "the relations between nurses and physicians are very good" (Level I). However, her Level II reponse is *true* — she thinks a physician would say that relations *are* very good. Her Level III response is also *true*, indicating she thinks that a physician would expect her to agree that relations are very good. To summarize, the nurse's response indicates that she does not believe that relations between the two professions are "very good." However, she does not think that a physician would *agree* with her (Level II), and she does not think that he *understands* her perception (Level III).

This configuration yields eight possible ways in which an item may be answered, as shown in Figure 3-2 with data from a preliminary survey of nurses. Figure 3-2 shows that there were 38 individuals who responded to the item, 32 of them responding False to Level I and 6 responding True. Thus, most of the nurses

Figure 3-2 Illustration of Possible Patterns of Answers to an Item of the IPS

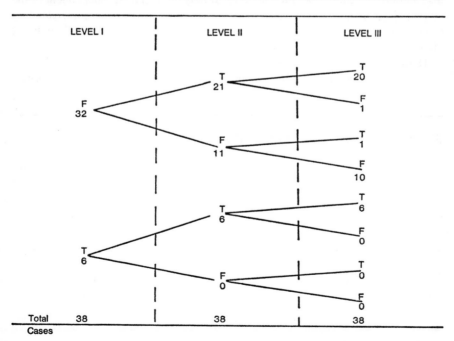

LEVEL I	LEVEL II	LEVEL III
		T 20
	T 21	
		F 1
F 32		
	F 11	T 1
		F 10
		T 6
	T 6	
		F 0
T 6		
	F 0	T 0
		F 0
Total 38	38	38
Cases		

who responded say that relations between nurses and physicians are not very good. If we continue to follow the responses of the 32 who answered False at Level I, we see that 21 of them say that physicians would indicate that relations are very good. In other words, two-thirds of the nurses who think relations are not good feel that physicians would perceive it differently. Interestingly enough however, about one-third of those who think that relations are not good think that physicians would agree with them. Furthermore, 10 of these nurses also believe that a physician would think that nurses would say relations were not good.

This method of analysis, by itself or coupled with the corresponding pattern from another profession, can yield a great deal of data concerning the way in which professions view their interrelationships. In this instance, from one profession's point of view we can see: how the nurse pictures the physician, how the nurse thinks the physician views himself, and how the nurse thinks the physician thinks she perceives him. Thus Level I responses yield a direct view of how one profession perceives another, but Level II and III responses yield additional data on whether one profession thinks the other agrees or disagrees with that direct perception, and whether the other profession understands or misunderstands that perception.

If the eight possible patterns of answers are placed in a two-by-two contingency table, the possibilities for analysis become more apparent. Figure 3-3 shows the distribution of the eight possible patterns. It may be seen that, independent of the direct perspective, one may perceive the other profession as either understanding or not understanding, and as either agreeing or not agreeing with one's point of view.

These patterns may also be examined in conjunction with one another. For example, the perceptions of physical therapists and special education teachers may

Figure 3-3 Possible Patterns of IPS Responses

	Perceived agreement	Perceived disagreement
Perceived understanding	T T T F F F	T F T F T F
Perceived misunderstanding	T T F F F T	T F F F T T

be compared. Thus it is possible to develop a view of the total pattern of perceptions between two or more professions.

The Initial Scale

The initial version of the Interprofessional Perception Scale consisted of 25 items concerned with professional issues such as competence, ethics, trust, status, and autonomy. A pilot study using this scale was conducted with a group of 38 nurses who were enrolled in the masters level course in nursing practice.

Results of the pilot study indicate that there are some areas where the nurses in the sample perceived the physicians' perceptions as different from their own. These differences center primarily on perceptions of ethical standards, welfare of the patient, and relationships between the nurse and the physician. The nurses do not perceive differences in perceptions of the physicians' status, competence, or importance to the health care team; however, there is some question regarding the physicians' knowledge of the capabilities of nurses.

The impact of such a pattern on the operation of the interdisciplinary team is indirect. For example, the results suggest that it may appear to some nurses that they are the patients' advocate in securing and utilizing the competence of the physician. It would seem that additional information regarding the mutual perceptions of various professionals involved in interdisciplinary teamwork would be helpful in further studying the operation of the team. For this reason the authors undertook a revision of the Interprofessional Perception Scale.

Development of the Refined Scale (IPS)

On the basis of the results from the preliminary instrument discussed above, it was possible to eliminate a number of items that were either redundant or contained ambiguities. For example, an item that stated "the relationship between nurses and physicians could be characterized as an uneasy truce," proved difficult to interpret and was eliminated. Fifteen items were included in the second version of the instrument. These items were reworded and the format and directions changed so that the IPS could be used with any pair of professions. Instructions for the revised form of the IPS may be found in Figure 3-4. The IPS form used for *other professions* is found in Figure 3-5, and Figure 3-6 shows the form used for measuring perceptions of one's *own profession* and how it is thought to be perceived by others.

Content validity of the instrument is established by the direct nature of the questions posed. Reliability was established through a test-retest procedure over a three-week period, using the responses of 24 students in a graduate rehabilitation counseling program. Using scales for physicians, social workers, and "own profession," the reliabilities as measured by percent of exact agreement ranged from 74 percent to 86 percent for Level I responses, with a mean across professions of 80 percent. Level II measures showed a range of reliabilities of 74 percent to 81 percent, with a mean of 79 percent. Level III reliabilities were 72 percent to 80 percent with a mean of 74 percent. Slightly lower reliabilities had been predicted for Level III in view of the complexity of the response (How would other professionals say you answered?).

Figure 3-4 Interprofessional Perception Scale

All answers are confidential. *Do not sign this form.*

Respondent data: Profession _____

Age _____ Sex _____   Years Experience _____

Highest Degree or
  Certificate _____   Specialty
                                                   (if applicable) _____

This is a study of interprofessional perceptions. It is intended to get at some of the ways various professions view each other and how they think others view them.

Please fill in the information at the top of this page, but *do not sign your name.*

In answering the following items, do not spend too much time on any one statement. Your first impression is what we want. Please answer with as much candor as possible. Answer all three parts of each question as you proceed. Each page should take only about 5 minutes. *Please answer each item.*

As you look at the following page, you will see that in Column 1 you should indicate whether you think the statement is true or false; in Column II you should indicate how you think the other professional would answer; and in Column III, how you think they would predict you would answer. Please place an X to indicate your answers.

You may begin now.

Figure 3-5 Interprofessional Perception Scale

Answer the following items in relation to this profession:

Physical Therapy

Persons in this profession:	How Would You Answer?		How Would They Answer?		How Would They Say That You Answered?	
	TRUE	FALSE	TRUE	FALSE	TRUE	FALSE
1. Are competent	☐	☐	☐	☐	☐	☐
2. Have very little autonomy	☐	☐	☐	☐	☐	☐
3. Understand the capabilities of your profession	☐	☐	☐	☐	☐	☐
4. Are highly concerned with the welfare of the patient	☐	☐	☐	☐	☐	☐
5. Sometimes encroach on your professional territory	☐	☐	☐	☐	☐	☐
6. Are highly ethical	☐	☐	☐	☐	☐	☐
7. Expect too much of your profession	☐	☐	☐	☐	☐	☐
8. Have a higher status than your profession	☐	☐	☐	☐	☐	☐
9. Are very defensive about their professional prerogatives	☐	☐	☐	☐	☐	☐
10. Trust your professional judgment	☐	☐	☐	☐	☐	☐
11. Seldom ask your professional advice	☐	☐	☐	☐	☐	☐
12. Fully utilize the capabilities of your profession	☐	☐	☐	☐	☐	☐
13. Do not cooperate well with your profession	☐	☐	☐	☐	☐	☐
14. Are well trained	☐	☐	☐	☐	☐	☐
15. Have good relations with your profession	☐	☐	☐	☐	☐	☐

Figure 3-6 Interprofessional Perception Scale

Answer the following items in relation to <u>Your Own Profession</u>

Persons in this profession:	How Would You Answer?		How Would Other Health Professionals Answer?		How Would Other Health Professionals Say You Answered?	
	TRUE	FALSE	TRUE	FALSE	TRUE	FALSE
1. Are competent	☐	☐	☐	☐	☐	☐
2. Have very little autonomy	☐	☐	☐	☐	☐	☐
3. Understand the capabilities of other professions	☐	☐	☐	☐	☐	☐
4. Are highly concerned with the welfare of the patient	☐	☐	☐	☐	☐	☐
5. Sometimes encroach on other professional territories	☐	☐	☐	☐	☐	☐
6. Are highly ethical	☐	☐	☐	☐	☐	☐
7. Expect too much of other professions	☐	☐	☐	☐	☐	☐
8. Have a higher status than other professions	☐	☐	☐	☐	☐	☐
9. Are very defensive about their professional prerogatives	☐	☐	☐	☐	☐	☐
10. Trust others' professional judgments	☐	☐	☐	☐	☐	☐
11. Seldom ask others' professional advice	☐	☐	☐	☐	☐	☐
12. Fully utilize the capabilities of other professions	☐	☐	☐	☐	☐	☐
13. Do not cooperate well with other professions	☐	☐	☐	☐	☐	☐
14. Are well trained	☐	☐	☐	☐	☐	☐
15. Have good relations with other professions	☐	☐	☐	☐	☐	☐

Results of Revised IPS

In a preliminary study of the revised instrument, scales measuring perceptions of physicians, nurses, and own profession were administered to 29 allied health professionals. The subjects included physical therapists (n=9), medical technologists (n=9), nutritionists (n=5), respiratory therapists (n=2), and one each of occupational therapist, child care worker, social worker, and unidentified affiliation. Each subject was asked to complete the 15-item scale for physicians, nurses, and own profession for each of the three response levels, yielding 135 items. The data were analyzed for each profession and for each response level, using Fisher's Exact Test.

The results indicate that there were significant relationships between levels of response in 58 of 109 possible instances (26 instances were not calculated due to the absence of data in two or more cells). In general, there was an association between the subjects' view of the other profession (Level I) and the subjects' perception of how the profession viewed themselves (Level II). Among the items in which the allied health professionals perceived disagreement and misunderstanding with both nurses and physicians were the following: understanding the capabilities of other professionals, encroaching on professional territory, defensiveness about professional prerogatives, and not utilizing fully the capabilities of other professions. Items that indicated potential disagreement and misunderstanding with other professionals regarding one's own profession included: concern with the welfare of the patient, expectations of other professions, asking professional advice, and trusting the professional judgments of others.

Looking at the Level I responses provides some interesting perspectives of allied health professionals concerning physicians and nurses. For instance, only 13.8 percent of the subjects felt that nurses understood the capabilities of the allied health professions. The comparable figure for physicians is 10.3 percent. As to utilization of the capabilities of the allied health professional, only 20.7 percent of the respondents indicated that nurses did so fully (6.9 percent for physicians). On the other hand, respondents indicated that physicians are competent (85.7 percent), highly ethical (67.9 percent), and have good relations with their profession (75.0 percent). The comparable figures for nurses are 75.9 percent, 67.9 percent, and 48.3 percent.

In general, the subjects appeared to think that both nurses and physicians were competent and well trained, but did not realize or fully utilize the capabilities of the various allied health professionals. An examination of responses at Level II and Level III indicates that many of the subjects did not think that nurses or physicians agree with or understand their perspective on these issues. For example, as noted above, only 10.3 percent of the respondents indicated that physicians understand the capabilities of their profession, but 86.2 percent said that physicians would indicate that they *did* understand those capabilities. Similarly, 75.9 percent of the subjects said that physicians would expect them to respond *yes* to that item.

A second study was conducted, using a sample of 115 health professionals including nurses, physical therapists, special educators, rehabilitation counselors, and others. Responses to some selected items are of interest. Table 3-1 reveals the response to the item "Persons in this profession are competent."

Table 3-1 Persons in This Profession Are Competent

Percent of "True" Responses from a Sample of 115 * Health Professions

Profession	Level I How would you answer?	Level II How would they answer?	Level III How would they say you answered?
Nursing N=86	81.4	98.8	88.4
Physical Therapy N=51	100	100	96.1
Medicine (Physician) N=110	89.1	89.1	96.4
Social Work N=81	81.5	100	87.7

*Not all individuals were asked to respond to each of the other professions, therefore the Ns differ.

As may be seen from the data, there is a high level of agreement that persons in these fields are indeed competent. (It should be noted that no person answered this question concerning their own profession, that question being in another questionnaire). More than 80 percent of the respondents in each instance indicated that they thought the other profession was indeed competent. For the most part the respondents believe the other professions would answer that they are competent, and that others would say the same about them. The item concerning ethics shows a similar pattern, however the percentage of true answers at Level I is somewhat lower. The question of professional ethics (Table 3-2) is one of great concern, and it is surprising that in the cases of social work, nursing, and medicine, more than 25 percent of the sample do not see those professionals as being highly ethical.

Table 3-2 Persons in This Profession Are Highly Ethical

Percent of "True" Responses from a Sample of 115* Health Professionals

Profession	Level I How would you answer?	Level II How would they answer?	Level III How would they say you answered?
Nursing N=85	74.1	94.2	88.4
Physical Therapy N=51	88.2	92.2	96.1
Medicine (Physician) N=51	74.5	95.5	86.4
Social Work N=79	69.6	96.2	86.1

*Not all individuals were asked to respond to each of the other professions; therefore the Ns differ.

Another area that affects the functioning of the interdisciplinary team is professional territoriality. The data indicate that our sample did indeed see the four professions they were questioned about as encroaching on their territory to some degree. In the case of physicians, the pattern is interesting. Over 70 percent indicated encroachment, and less than 20 percent said the physician would say this (Table 3-3).

Teamwork depends on the full utilization of the competency of individual team members. Full use of the capabilities of each profession might be assumed to enhance the effectiveness of the team. Table 3-4 indicates that most of the sample did not perceive other professionals made full use of their capabilities.

Table 3-3 Persons in This Profession Sometimes Encroach on Your Professional Territory

Percent of "True" Responses from a Sample of 115* Health Professionals

Profession	Level I How would you answer?	Level II How would they answer?	Level III How would they say you answered?
Nursing N=85	54.1	10.6	29.4
Physical Therapy N=51	31.4	19.6	37.3
Medicine (Physician) N=111	72.1	17.1	38.7
Social Work N=81	54.3	22.2	46.9

*Not all individuals were asked to respond to each of the other professions; therefore the Ns differ.

Table 3-4 Persons in This Profession Fully Utilize the Capabilities of Your Profession

Percent of "True" Responses from a Sample of 115* Health Professions

Profession	Level I How would you answer?	Level II How would they answer?	Level III How would they say you answered?
Nursing N=87	21.8	59.8	46.0
Physical Therapy N=51	23.5	54.9	43.1
Medicine (Physician) N=111	15.3	73.6	60.9
Social Work N=79	36.7	82.3	60.8

*Not all individuals were asked to respond to each of the other professions; therefore the Ns differ.

Table 3-5 represents a somewhat different perspective in that it shows how the sample perceives their own professions. For example, almost 90 percent of the respondents said that persons in their own profession were competent, but indicated that they think about 77 percent of other health professionals would agree with this assessment. The item asking whether the sample fully utilizes the capabilities of other professions is of interest when compared to Table 3-4.

These results are indeed preliminary, and care must be exercised in drawing firm conclusions at this point. Still it is clear that many of these areas deserve further investigation.

Table 3-5 Reactions to Questions Concerning Their Own Professions

Percent of "True" Responses from a Sample of 115* Health Professionals

Persons in this profession:	How would you answer?	How would other health professionals answer?	How would other health professionals say you answered?
Are competent N=112	89.3	76.8	97.3
Are highly ethical N=111	88.3	79.3	90.9
Sometimes encroach on other professional territories N=113	55.6	61.9	41.6
Fully utilize the capabilities of other professions N=111	53.6	47.3	62.6

*Not all individuals responded to this portion of the instrument.

The preliminary studies suggest that the IPS may be a promising technique for the systematic measurement of interprofessional perceptions. The early findings suggest that the instrument might help to identify areas of disagreement and misunderstanding between professions and indicate areas of potential conflict within interdisciplinary teams. The information provided at the three response levels could also be useful in the education of health care professionals. For example, if information is available concerning how a profession such as physical therapy is perceived by others, students can be prepared to deal with those perceptions in a realistic way. The instrument can also be used to monitor the effects of specific curricular components on the interprofessional perceptions of students. The instrument could even be used as a point of departure in interdisciplinary education to show various professionals how they view one another and explore the reasons for such perceptions. Further research on interprofessional perceptions is needed before we can fully understand the relationships between team members and the impact of these relationships on team effectiveness.

PROFESSIONAL ETHICS

One of the major functions of the professional association is the development of a code of ethics designed to regulate the conduct of its members. As previously noted, society awards considerable autonomy to the profession and its members, with the understanding that this freedom will not be abused. A code of ethics ensures that this autonomy is not misused. By providing clearcut guidelines on appropriate and inappropriate behaviors in relation to colleagues and clients, the professional association attempts to control or modify the actions of its members. Although initially some codes may be, as Sussman (1966) suggests, "an imprecise compilation of well-intentioned statements defining professional conduct" (p. 192), as the profession matures the code is refined and elaborated. However, even in its early stages, a profession's code of ethical standards indicates the normative professional behaviors expected of its members and thus has some implications for interprofessional relationships and the team approach. Team members may view situations quite differently as a result of differing value systems, and an ethical code might be expected to reflect those values generally accepted within a particular profession.

In order to look at the interdisciplinary implications of such standards, the ethical codes of 20 representative health professions were examined (Golin and Ducanis, 1977). The professional associations included in the study are listed in Table 3-6. Although many of the codes include additional interpretive statements, this discussion is limited to the codes themselves.

A preliminary examination of the codes revealed five major topics covered by the ethical guidelines: professional competence, relationships with colleagues, relationships with clients, legal responsibilities, and responsibilities to society. These topics were then used to categorize every statement in the 20 codes. In several codes, each statement was already numbered; in the others, paragraphs or sentences that seemed to express a single integral idea were numbered by the authors. This process yielded a total of 468 identified statements which were then coded in the five categories. Each statement was coded only once; however, the categories were not mutually exclusive, so that some statements contained reference to more than one category. For example, statements dealing with the referral of clients to other colleagues might be categorized either as category II (clients), or III (colleagues). In such cases, coding was based on what appeared to be the dominant theme, but this was a subjective judgment of the authors. After this initial coding, the statements were further sorted into subcategories. Figure 3-7 presents the five major categories and their subcategories.

Table 3-6 Twenty Professional Associations Sampled

1. American Association for Respiratory Therapy
2. American College of Hospital Administrators
3. American Dental Assistants Association
4. American Dental Association
5. American Dental Hygienists Association
6. American Dietetic Association
7. American Medical Association
8. American Medical Record Association
9. American Medical Technologists
10. American Nurses Association
11. American Occupational Therapy Association
12. American Optometric Association
13. American Personnel and Guidance Association
14. American Physical Therapy Association
15. American Podiatry Association
16. American Psychological Association
17. American Society for Medical Technology
18. American Speech and Hearing Association
19. National Association of Social Workers
20. National Rehabilitation Counseling Association

Figure 3-7 Categories and Subcategories of Twenty Ethical Codes

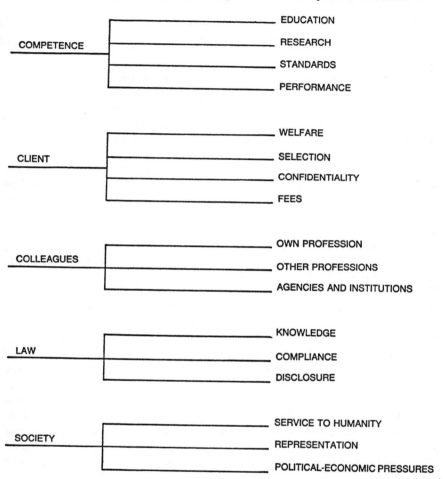

Professional Competence

The largest number of statements (128) were classified under the category of professional competence. This category includes statements on professional knowledge and skills. Subcategories of this topic are: education, professional standards, performance, and research.

Three major aspects of education are stressed: initial preparation, continuing education, and the exchange of knowledge between professionals. There is no discernible disagreement among the various codes concerning the importance of these factors; what does differ is the level of specificity concerning the individual's responsibility in these areas. Some codes include only a brief sentence of what is expected while others contain a much more detailed description.

Along with requirements for continuing education, review and evaluation of the competence of members is also mentioned. In addition, a number of codes mention the need to practice the profession in a manner meeting the highest professional standards. There appears to be no disagreement among the professions in regard to the principle of maintenance of high standards of performance; however there may be some potential for conflict in the enforcement of these standards.

The personal conduct of the individual in the performance of his professional role is considered in almost all of the codes. Such considerations as personal honesty, the boundaries of professional practice, and factors that may interfere with the performance of one's professional duties are included within this subcategory. For example, one code states, "No member shall endeavor to extend his province beyond his competence and the authority invested to him by a physician" (American Association for Respiratory Therapy, undated).

Factors interfering with adequate performance may be either internal (such as personal problems) or external (such as factors related to the employment situation). While the codes are in general agreement in the area of performance, there seems to be one point of potential controversy — in the limits or boundaries which each profession either imposes on itself or has imposed on it. As professions develop, they tend to carve out areas of practice, sometimes at the expense of older, more established professions. Such attempts to broaden the limits of practice may indeed lead to interprofessional conflicts. Certainly when the boundaries are spelled out in written codes, the professional may feel quite justified in opposing any encroachment of territory by others and may condemn their actions as "unethical."

The attention given to ethical concerns about research activities varies greatly by profession. As expected, those professional groups less involved in direct research are not as likely to specify regulations for research activities as are psychology and medicine, fields that are more research oriented. In general, those codes dealing with research express the need for further research, voice a concern for the welfare of human subjects, and devote attention to the problems of informed consent and confidentiality.

Responsibilities to Clients

The second major category identified in Figure 3-7 contained 105 statements dealing with individuals, organizations, and groups receiving professional services. These included statements referring to the welfare of the client, how clients may be selected, questions of confidentiality of client information, and the setting of fees. In this category, those statements dealing with confidentiality and disclosure of information seem potentially to have the greatest impact on team functioning since the codes vary greatly in their approach to this question. While the codes generally agree concerning the need to disclose information in order to protect the client or the community, only one of the 20 codes refers specifically to the need to share information with the team (although it is also mentioned in the interpretive statements of another profession). In general, the codes require the professional to "respect," "guard," and/or "protect" the patient's rights of privacy and confidentiality. According to one code, the right of confidentiality also extends to professional communication, which cannot be shared with the individual involved unless express permission is given by the originator. As Banta and Fox (1972) reported, a serious problem of communication can arise when members of an interprofessional team hold different views regarding the sharing of confidential information. Of course, open communication is the basis of the team approach, but the ambiguity in the codes on this point suggests that many professionals do not have clearcut professional guidelines concerning what they can share with team members. It is not clear how some of these issues will be resolved as the team approach becomes more widespread.

Other topics in this category include prohibitions against solicitation of patients and discrimination in patient selection, regulations about the setting of fees, and general statements regarding protecting the welfare of the client.

Responsibilities to Colleagues

The third category contains 119 statements dealing with relationships with colleagues of one's own profession, of other professions, and with various agencies and organizations. Many of these statements focus on the need for professional cooperation and thus have real implications for the interdisciplinary team. Guidelines regarding intraprofessional relationships include statements referring to professional associations, consultation and referral practices, and the professional's responsibility to report unethical or incompetent behavior to the professional association or other appropriate agency. Such action could obviously have widespread repercussions and could lead to many problems. On the other hand, failure to act is inconsistent with the notion of responsibility for the welfare of the client.

In many of the statements concerning relationships with other professions, the focus is on interprofessional "cooperation" and "harmony." One code refers specifically to interdisciplinary teamwork, and instructs that when *team* decisions are involved, the professional will "abide by and help to implement those decisions even though he might not personally agree with them" (National Rehabilitation Counseling Association, 1972). The need to be familiar with the practices and competencies of other professions is also mentioned in a few codes, but for the most part the requirements of cooperation are expressed in rather general, somewhat ambiguous terms. Some professionals are enjoined by their ethical standards to treat the views of others with "respect" and to avoid "encroachment."

The professional is held responsible for the actions of others, and even when faced with the incompetent or unethical behavior of those outside his or her own profession, the professional is obligated to attempt to rectify the situation.

Relationships with employing agencies and institutions are discussed in terms of "loyalty" and "support." However, this does not necessarily extend to condoning all policies of the institution, and several codes clearly indicate an ethical responsibility to attempt to change poor conditions. For example, from social work comes the following statement:

> I accept responsibility for working toward the creation and *maintainance (sic)* of conditions within agencies that enable social workers to conduct themselves in keeping with this code (National Association of Social Workers, 1967).

And from psychology:

> As employees of an institution or agency, psychologists have the responsibility of remaining alert to and attempting to mediate institutional pressures that may distort reports of psychological findings or impede their proper use (American Psychological Association, 1977).

It is interesting that in these statements dealing with professional colleagues and agencies, there is very little explicit attention given to the question of professional autonomy. Autonomy would seem to be a major element in professionalization, particularly in regard to relations between professions, but the professional is given little or no specific guidance in this area. If the team approach continues as a major force in the delivery of human services, it seems likely that increasing attention will be given to the potential problems in this area.

Legal Responsibility

This category includes 19 statements referring to legal constraints that regulate the professional's activities. These included statements about knowledge of the law, compliance with the law, and disclosure of the illegal acts of others. It can be expected that in the future there will be considerably more attention given to this area, as the legal ramifications of the delivery of health care and related services become more numerous and complex. In fact, some of the new legislation dealing with patients' rights might make parts of present ethical guides obsolete.

Responsibilities to Society

The final category includes 97 statements referring to the professional's relationships with the public-at-large and how the profession itself is represented to the public. Included here are a number of statements such as that of the AMA: "The principle objective of the medical profession is to render service to humanity with full respect for the dignity of man" (American Medical Association, 1971). Similarly, "the dentist has the obligation of providing freely of his skills, knowledge and experience to society" (American Dental Association, 1976). The associations show a great deal of concern with their image and how they are represented by their members, as well as how professionals present themselves to the public and the means used to notify potential clients of available services. Finally, the professional is warned against yielding to various political and/or economic pressures, and in several codes is expressly enjoined against conflicts of interest or the use of rebates. Generally it would appear that those sections of the codes dealing with social and legal matters have less obvious implications for team functioning.

Questions for the Future

A number of questions regarding the ethical guidelines of professional groups and the interdisciplinary team come to mind after reviewing the 20 codes:

1. Should the guidelines be uniform across professions that are expected to work together closely?
2. To what extent are the guidelines actually enforced? Do they in fact represent a "paper tiger"?
3. Are the ethical guidelines as presently written conducive to teamwork or do they actually hinder interdisciplinary endeavors?
4. Are the various standards too protective of professional autonomy and separateness, and are they sometimes used as an excuse for noncooperative behavior?

5. Should professions be trained in the ethical standards of other professions as well as their own? Would this help avoid interprofessional conflicts?
6. What impact will changes in legislation (such as that concerned with patient rights) and changes in funding patterns (such as third party payment plans) have on the ethical standards of the profession?

It is still too early for definitive answers to these questions. Only with more experience in team functionings will the role of the professional organizations and their ethical codes be clarified. However, it appears that we can probably expect a number of changes with regard to the ethical standards of the various professions as we move through marked changes in the human service delivery system.

Chapter 4

The Client

There are several reasons for using a team approach in providing services to individuals. Among them is a growing realization that any one profession simply does not encompass a sufficient knowledge base to deal adequately with complex human problems. The team approach is one way to integrate the skills and knowledge of several specialists. Specialities and subspecialities sometimes treat various human ills as though one aspect of the individual has no connection to any other. The problem this poses has been clear to most human service professionals for some time; however, the solution is still elusive. This chapter examines the role of the client in the treatment process and how the client and the team may interact.

THE PRESENTING PROBLEM

Clients usually referred to an interdisciplinary team have one or more specific problems which the team is expected to alleviate. The unique set of problems presented by each client defines the task of the team and determines which professional skills are required to adequately serve the client.

This principle is illustrated by the following case study of a hypothetical client seen in the rehabilitation unit of a large metropolitan hospital.

Case Study 1

Johnny is a 20-year-old white male who was hospitalized two months ago with a spinal cord injury suffered in a motorcycle accident. Johnny lives in a rural area of western Pennsylvania and was recently transferred to this rehabilitation unit from the hospital near his home where he was treated following the accident.

Johnny's parents are living and his father is receiving disability payments as the result of a coal mining accident four years ago. Johnny has four brothers and three sisters, all older than he. Three of his brothers are working in the mines, and the fourth moved to California several years ago and is employed as a trucker. The sisters are all married and living nearby.

Johnny quit school in the 11th grade and has been employed as a construction worker for the last two years. He has been married for six months to Alice, whom he has known since high school. Although they had dated briefly a few years ago, they had not become serious about one another until they began dating again last December. Alice is now three and a half months pregnant and because of Johnny's accident is seriously considering an abortion.

Since being transferred to the rehabilitation unit, Johnny has been severely withdrawn with periods of angry acting out. The nurses report that he uses abusive language and constantly complains about the "service in this lousy hotel." The physical therapist indicates that he refuses to cooperate and tells her that he just wants to be left alone.

Johnny has not regained feeling or movement in his lower limbs and the outlook for recovery of function below the injury site is poor. He has a recurrent catheter infection which has been of concern, although at present it seems to be under control.

In this case we see that Johnny presents a number of present and future problems in addition to the trauma of physical injury. A rather large interdisciplinary team would be needed to adequately cope with his case. The professionals involved in Johnny's recovery might include, in addition to the physician and nursing staff, a physical therapist, an occupational therapist, an activities of-daily-living (ADL) worker, a psychologist, a social worker, a rehabilitation counselor, and a dietitian. A surgical team may have been required shortly after the accident, and another team of professionals may become involved in home care after his discharge from the hospital. In addition to treating Johnny's physical condition, appropriate team members might also deal with his emotional adjustments to the disability, the problems encountered by the family, Johnny's future vocational plans and economic circumstances, and the accommodations necessary in his living quarters when he returns home. It is apparent that no one profession encompasses all of the skills necessary to cope with all of these problems.

Now let us look at another client who might be seen at the outpatient unit of an alcohol and drug treatment center.

Case Study 2

Mr. Al J. is a 43-year-old white male who works as an insurance salesman. He is self-referred to this agency, having called for an appointment at the insistence of his wife, following a weekend of heavy drinking.

The client has been married for 22 years and has three children: Allen, Jr., age 21; Elizabeth, age 18; and Jeffrey, age 16. The older son is attending a state university about 100 miles from his home; the daughter is attending secretarial school and living at home. The younger son is a sophomore in high school. He has been having some problems lately and has been referred to juvenile court for shoplifting and truancy.

Mr. J. has been in his present job for 10 years and was previously employed in a similar job with another company for 14 years. He left that situation because of friction with his immediate supervisor. Although his work record at the present company is generally good, he has recently missed some important appointments and has been warned by his sales manager to "straighten out."

His wife has never worked outside the home since their marriage, but has recently enrolled in a refresher course in clerical and typing skills and is beginning to talk about looking for a job. Mr. J. is very disturbed by this and feels she should stay home to take care of their younger son.

In the initial intake interview, the client revealed that he has decided to seek treatment at this time primarily because his wife has threatened to leave him unless he stops drinking. Mr. J. denies he is an alcoholic but thinks he may have a problem with his drinking from time to time. However, he blames his drinking on stresses at home and his wife's "nagging." On the other hand, he says he loves her and does not want her to leave him.

The immediate problems presented by Mr. J. concern the physical and psychological effects of his drinking. However, there are a number of related difficulties, such as his job and marital problems and his son's trouble with the law, that are also significant aspects of the total picture. An appropriate team to deal with these problems might include a physician to assess the extent of physical damage and provide medical supervision for detoxification (if necessary), an alcohol counselor or therapist to provide individual and/or group counseling, and a social worker to work with the family. Thus the nature and extent of the presenting problems help determine the size and type of team that is needed.

A somewhat different picture is presented by another hypothetical client and the educational team providing services to her.

Case Study 3

Jane R. is a 15-year-old high school student who is congenitally blind. Jane is of average intelligence and is generally in good health, but has some speech difficulties in addition to her visual impairment. She and her family have recently moved to a suburban community outside the city where they had previously resided, and Jane will attend the public high school a few blocks from her home. Jane is being evaluated by personnel in her new school for educational planning for the coming year. Her parents have been asked to attend a team meeting for the development of an individualized educational program (IEP) for Jane.

The educational team serving Jane is likely to include a regular classroom teacher, a special education teacher of the visually handicapped, the school psychologist who is now evaluating Jane, the speech therapist who will work with Jane's speech problems, and perhaps the school principal. Jane's parents are expected to play an important role in the team decision making, and Jane herself may be asked to participate in the development of the IEP.

Jane's special education teacher may also coordinate a number of resources outside the school. Medical records from the ophthalmologist may be needed; a volunteer Braillist may be required to transcribe some of Jane's work into Braille; other volunteers may be used to tape record reading material for her; and Jane may be referred to a counselor from the State Office for the Blind for vocational rehabilitation services.

In the meantime, the IEP team will begin concrete educational planning for Jane in order to determine the overall goals and specific objectives for the coming year, as well as spell out how these objectives might be met. These plans might include the further development of Jane's academic skills, orientation and mobility training for the new environment, and speech therapy to improve Jane's oral expression.

Thus we see again how the problems presented by the individual client structures the way in which the team will work with the client and even determines who will be involved in the team approach.

CLIENT-TEAM INTERACTION

Although the presenting problems are of major importance in structuring the interaction of the client and the team, other characteristics of the client also influence this interaction. Each client has a number of traits that do not necessarily relate directly to the problem that led the client to seek the help of the team. Age, sex, intelligence, personality, and cultural background all influence the way in which the client and the team will interact. For example, the impact of age on such interaction is illustrated in a study of the attitudes of stroke patients toward the hospital in which they received initial care (Christie and Lawrence, 1978). The authors conclude that:

> Attitudes towards the hospital experience were observed to be age-related in both men and women. . . . Reasons for this can only be speculative in the context of the present study. Stroke often brings major change into people's lives and to men especially, the threat includes not only loss of status within the family, but also downgrading of occupation or forced retirement. With older men these threats are more likely to materialize and it is not difficult to understand their resentment of enforced dependency and of the young, mostly male doctors. As women grow older they seem to fit more easily into a dependent role (p. 51).

Not only were client attitudes affected by attributes such as age, the behavior of the professionals was also affected. Christie and Lawrence conclude that "the pattern appearing throughout this study is that in an age of high technology the ability, or willingness, of many professionals to talk with and understand people who are old, infirm, or 'difficult' because they can't speak English, is sadly lacking in all too many cases" (p. 51). As we noted in Chapter One, the way in which the client and the team interact is a product of the characteristics of the client, the professionals on the team, and the organizational setting in which the encounter occurs.

Although the client is frequently seen as a passive recipient of the team's efforts rather than as an active participant in the team, the client plays a crucial role in the treatment process. First of all, the client has an intimate acquaintance with the problem either on an intellectual basis or on the basis of past experience. Second, their cooperation is necessary if treatment is to be successful. Third, they generally have more reason to be concerned about their welfare than any other person. Finally, it is generally the client who will make (or should make) the final decision concerning treatment or nontreatment.

The interdisciplinary team must deal with the client differently than when the therapeutic situation is primarily a dyadic "doctor-patient" relationship. Although the professionals may be expert in only a few aspects of the client's needs, they nevertheless must be *concerned* with all aspects of the client. Comprehensive care requires that the team deal with the client as a totality. This is not to say that the team will not emphasize one or another aspect of need at a particular time, but rather that no aspect of the client's problem should be neglected.

We can identify four areas of client-team interaction: *seeking behavior* — in general, the team does not find the client, the client finds the team; *information giving* — the client informs the team of the problem through several modes, including giving a blood sample or "telling the doctor where it hurts"; *cooperation in treatment* — active involvement, not the passive role suggested by the term *compliance;* and *participation in the decision-making process* — an awareness of the possibilities and dangers of any diagnostic procedure or therapeutic regimen.

Seeking Behavior

It is part of the client's responsibility to enter the system. Although this seems like a simple statement, it is not to be taken lightly. In a democratic society clients do not have to enter the human service system unless they choose to or unless their condition or behavior constitutes a clear threat to society at large. Even then, the choice of whether to be *treated* in the system is still in the client's hands, except where the client is judged to be incompetent to make such a decision.

Thus children may be forced to attend school and some mental patients may be treated unwillingly, but the great majority of clients seek help voluntarily. Because of the importance of such seeking behavior, it has been the aim of many health screening and health education programs to activate such behavior on the part of individuals when certain signs or symptoms occur. Some seeking behavior is enforced by law, such as compulsory physical examinations for food service workers or teachers. Other seeking behavior is reinforced by social sanction, as when an employer reimburses employees for the expense of an annual physical examination or provides such examinations as part of the employee benefit package.

The client's willingness to seek help is influenced by a number of factors including the type and severity of the problem, the client's age and circumstances, and the availability of services. The client's usual mode of coping with stress may also affect seeking behavior. A middle-aged woman who discovers a lump in her breast through self-examination may quickly contact her physician for an examination, or she may deny the importance of the symptom and postpone seeking help, or she may become so frightened that she cannot face the problem and refuses any medical assistance. Attitudes toward the symptoms can also influence how clients react to problems. Thus the parents of a five-year-old boy will not hesitate to seek help if the child develops a sudden fever or other physical symptom, but may delay for several months seeking help when the child suddenly develops severe behavior problems.

Information Giving

The client is the prime source of information — indeed often the only source of information about himself. Others may add information, but only in relation to the client's actions or associations. Occasionally, others may have certain information that is not available to the client, such as the cause of death of parents or grandparents. The type of information given by the client is conditioned by factors such as ethnic background, sex, and age. Of course, the perceptions of the professional may be influenced by the same factors, and care must be taken to ensure that relevant information is not lost due to differences in the way information is imparted or received.

Cooperation in Treatment

In order to fulfill the client role the person must either submit to treatment or must actively take part in that treatment. Sometimes active participation may mean only allowing the procedures to be performed; however, generally there is a need for the client to "do" something. If there is one area in the medical literature that resounds with frustration, it is that which deals with *compliance,* that is, the client's ability or willingness to follow a prescribed treatment regimen. Changing human habits is a difficult task, and it is no less difficult for those in the health care professions. For example, look at the number of people who continue to smoke in the face of all evidence, warnings, and symptoms that point to the dangers involved. The degree of client cooperation in treatment has long been a subject of intense concern among health professionals.

Participation in the Decision-Making Process

In most cases, people have the right to decide for themselves what they wish to do with their bodies and even their lives. This concept is difficult for many professionals to accept, since they have, by training and experience, come to expect that once a client has appeared, he or she will follow whatever advice or "orders" are given by the professional. Currently, however, it seems that many clients are moving toward a more active role in making decisions concerning their treatment. Several factors have influenced this trend.

First, there has been an increased general *awareness* of health care among the public as a result of various newspaper and magazine articles, books, television shows, and movies that have dealt with health-related topics.

Second, the impact of the *consumer movement* on health care and human services has been significant. There have been dramatic changes in the area of patient rights and rights of the handicapped. Judicial rulings and legislative mandates have supported the consumer of human services.

Third, and perhaps most important, the general rise in the *educational level* of the population means that individuals are more knowledgeable, and in some cases more skeptical, about the services they receive.

Since the role of the client or patient is so crucial to team functioning let us examine more closely some of the ways that role has been viewed.

THE SICK ROLE

The concept of a sick "role" was articulated by Talcott Parsons in 1951. Illness was seen by Parsons as a "state of disturbance in the 'normal' functioning of the total human individual, including both the state of the organism as a biological system and of his personal and social adjustments. It is thus partly biologically and partly socially defined" (Parsons, 1951, p. 431). Thus the behavior of the ill person is not only a medical issue but also a social-psychological event. Parsons' analysis deals with the doctor-patient relationship, but this approach has many implications for the other helping professions.

Parsons contended that being sick was not simply a "condition" but a *social role,* the test of this being "the existence of a set of institutionalized expectations and the corresponding sentiments and sanctions" (p. 436). Parsons set about describing these role expectations in some detail.

> There seem to be four aspects of the institutionalized expectation system relative to the sick role. First, is the exception from normal social role responsibilities, which of course is relative to the nature and severity of the illness. . . . The second closely related aspect is the institutionalized definition that the sick person cannot be expected by "pulling himself together" to get well by an act of decision or will. . . . He can't "help it". . . . The third element is the definition of the state of being ill as itself undesirable with its obligation to want to "get well". . . . Finally, the fourth closely related element is the obligation — in proportion to the severity of the condition, of course — to seek *technically competent* help, namely, in the most usual case, that of a physician and to *cooperate* with him in the process of trying to get well. It is here, of course, that the role of the sick person as patient becomes articulated with that of the physician in a complimentary role structure (Parsons, 1951, pp. 436- 437).

So the sick role, as conceived by Parsons, carries with it the right to be exempt from the usual social responsibilities and recognizes that the individual is not responsible for his illness. Sick persons can stay home from work, refuse to drive the nursery school carpool, or miss classes — with a clear recognition by all that it is "not their fault." Along with these privileges are two obligations: to wish to recover, and to seek competent help. Sick persons are not supposed to enjoy the role too much; the "secondary gain" or positive byproducts of being sick are restricted, and patients are supposed to try to get better.

Although the sick role is in some ways a deviant role, it differs from other forms of deviance in that the "sick person is not regarded as 'responsible' for his condition, 'he can't help it.' He may, of course, have carelessly exposed himself to danger of accident, but then once injured he cannot, for example, mend a fractured leg by 'will power' '' (Parsons, 1951, p. 440).

The Parsonian model has been very influential in the sociology of medicine, in rehabilitation, and in special education — particularly in reference to the relationship between client and professional, and the way in which the institutionalized expectations of each party in the relationship will shape their role behaviors. As Wilson and Bloom (1972) point out, even those who disagree with Parsons' analysis may accept the notion of social roles adopted by patient and professional. "At issue is not the question whether patterned expectations exist but, rather, the assumptions which different theoretical positions take about the nature of these expectations" (p. 316).

Parsons and Fox (1952) compared the role relationships of doctor-patient with those of parent-child, indicating the similarities between the dependence of the child and the position of the sick person. Assuming that "the role of the physician, in the more general sense, is psychotherapeutic" (p. 40), four major aspects of therapy that have relevance for the professional's role are identified:

1. *Permissiveness* — Patients are allowed to express their feelings, wishes, and fantasies.
2. *Support* — This involves "accepting [the patient] as a bona fide member of the therapeutic system because he is deemed worth helping" (p. 40).
   This permissive-supportive approach is balanced by two methods used to control the patient's behavior.
3. *Denial of reciprocity* — The doctor "will adhere scrupulously to a professional attitude" (p. 40), and does not reciprocate the emotional responsiveness of the patient. This allows physicians to maintain an "asymmetrical" relationship in which they are clearly in charge. Professional neutrality and distance are used to maintain the professional's superior position vis-à-vis the patient.
4. *Conditional rewards* — The physician "introduces conditional rewards (of which his approval is probably the most important) for the patient's good work in the therapeutic situation" (p. 44).

Thus the doctor motivates the patient to become well and rewards efforts in that direction; this is the basis of the physician's leverage with the patient. Since, according to Parsons, the sick role is a temporary form of deviance in which the affected individual is unable to fulfill normal social roles, there are pressures on the patient to return to a nondeviant state. The role of the therapist then, is to ensure that the patient gives up the deviant sick role and resumes the responsibilities that have been temporarily set aside. Since both of these roles are too important to be left to chance, they have become institutionalized with reciprocal expectation on the part of the two players. In this sense the doctor and his patient can be viewed as a social system.

As noted earlier, the Parsonian model of the sick role has been a major influence in the sociology of medicine. However, a number of authors (Gallagher, 1976; Gordon, 1966; Freidson, 1961; Segall, 1976; and Wilson, 1970) have pointed to the need for modification and/or expansion of the original model. As Gallagher notes, one of the questions that may be raised about the Parsonian concept is that it is "medico-centric" — that is, the physician is at the center of medical care. However, often the physician alone is unable to provide the needed care so that a number of other services may be called upon to treat the patient's illness. "These varied resources, medical and non-medical, hospital-based and community-based, expand and supplement the services which the doctor directly provides" (Gallagher, 1976, p. 212). Gallagher suggests that although Parsons indicates that the total hospital must provide the same trust and support that the physician does, "however much influence the doctor has in the individual doctor-patient relationship, it cannot be delegated or transferred very far in a chain of medical referral or a hospital hierarchy" (Gallagher, 1976, p. 213).

A similar point has been made by Wilson:

> The practitioner is less and less commonly a solo agent providing comprehensive aid; instead a coordinated team of health professionals is engaged in a joint approach to medical risks. This inevitably means that the pattern of "resocialization" in the classic doctor-patient framework cannot occur on the same terms. To emphasize only a single difference, the client being helped by a battery of professionals can hardly muster the intensity of trust (and dependency) that undergirds the growth of transference in a psychotherapeutic encounter between *a* patient and *a* physician (Wilson, 1970, p. 23).

Thus it is felt that Parsons does not seem to adequately account for medical care involving a team approach or a group of professionals focused on a single client.

In addition to the numbers and kinds of helpers involved in health care, Wilson notes two other areas that present problems for the Parsons model of the asymmetrical doctor-patient relationship: the *nature of the illness* (that is, chronic illness and long term disability may not fit the model), and the *characteristics of those who are to be helped* (that is, the client may be given preventive rather than therapeutic medicine or may be a group rather than an individual).

Gallagher also focuses attention on the same three "problematic areas" of the Parsonian model, indicating that it does not adequately account for chronic illness and disability, preventive care and maintenance, or the varied roles of physicians and medical settings. He indicates that Parsons presents both the earlier deviance model and a later adaptation model that views health "as the adaptive capacity of the human organism." While the deviance concept has made a major contribution in several areas, Gallagher feels that the adaptation model may also prove to be a fruitful approach.

Freidson (1961) discusses the difficulties inherent in understanding the doctor-patient relationship and suggests that Parsons' analysis is based on ideal expectations rather than actual behavior. He suggests also that Parsons' definition of the sick role is drawn from the physician's perspective rather than from the perspective of the patient, the nurse, or any of the other involved parties. The doctor-patient relationship is seen by Freidson as a compromise of "conflicting needs, demands and forces" (p. 189). As Wilson and Bloom summarize it, "in place of the mutuality and reciprocity dynamics of the Parsonian analysis, Freidson substitutes hostility, ambivalence, and conflict" (1972, p. 316). To understand such relationships, according to Freidson, we must look at the expectations of all the involved parties and the "social structure in which those perspectives are located" (1961, p. 191), as well as the situations in which the doctor and patient find themselves. Thus, "the model of the structure of the doctor-patient relationship must encompass two distinct social systems — a professional system containing the doctor and a lay system containing the patient" (p. 192). Using the referral mechanism as the point of departure Freidson discusses in some detail how the patient moves through the lay-referral and professional-referral systems in the course of diagnosis and treatment.

Another approach to the patient role in the treatment process has been developed by Suchman (1965), who identified five stages in the sequence of medical events as the patient moves through the medical care system. Beginning with a definition of "illness behavior" first proposed by Mechanic and Volkart (1961) as "the way in which symptoms are perceived, evaluated and acted upon by a person who recognizes some pain, discomfort, or other sign of organic malfunction," Suchman looked at illness behavior in terms of patterns in the "seeking, finding and carrying out of medical care" (p. 114). Suchman's five stages and the decisions involved in each are:

1. **Symptom Experience Stage.** A middle-aged man wakes up with a scratchy throat, a ten-year-old boy comes home from school flushed and feverish, or a housewife notices pain and stiffness in her back: these are examples of the symptom experience stage. This is the period in which the potential patient first becomes aware of symptoms of illness and decides that something is wrong. The physical experience of pain or discomfort, the individual's interpretation of that experience, and the emotional reaction to it are the major elements of this beginning stage. Once the person is aware of symptoms, some evaluation of these symptoms takes place as the individual (or individual's family) decides on the next step. The person may react by denying the symptoms or delaying further action or may accept the symptoms and move on to the next stage.

2. **Assumption of the Sick Role.** At this stage the individual seeks temporary "provisional validation" as a sick person. Family and friends may be asked to diagnose or evaluate the individual's condition and attest to the illness. Self-

medication may be tried if the symptoms are not too severe. The man with a sore throat decides to stay in bed, the young boy is given aspirin and orange juice by his mother, and the housewife lies down with a heating pad while her husband cooks dinner. In the latter two cases, if the mother and the husband do not accept the validity of the claim to the sick role, the boy and the housewife will not be relieved of their normal responsibilities. At this stage the individual must decide if he or she is sick and needs professional care.

3. **Medical Care Contact.** If the symptoms persist or become more severe, the individual is likely to formally enter the professional medical care system. Only the professional can offer authoritative validation of the sick role. Thus the patient or patient's family calls the doctor or goes to the clinic for further diagnostic evaluation. The decision to seek medical care is an important one, but "once the decision to seek care is made, the initial medical contact is fairly well routinized and offers little difficulty to the patient" (Suchman, 1965, pp. 127-128).

4. **Dependent Patient Role.** By deciding to seek treatment and entering the medical care system, the individual becomes a patient. At this point the patient must decide whether to give control to the doctor and follow treatment procedures. The extent to which this dependency creates problems for the individual will vary from patient to patient. For some patients the "secondary gain" involved in the dependency of the patient role may actually interfere with recovery; for others the dependency may be more unbearable than the illness itself. Many people in our society seem to find this stage particularly difficult to accept.

5. **Recovery and Rehabilitation.** The course of the patient's illness may be long or short, mild or severe. However, in most cases the patient will eventually relinquish the "sick" role and return to normal activities and responsibilities. The middle-aged man goes back to work, the young boy returns to school, and the housewife resumes her normal routine. The decision to give up the patient role normally marks this stage. But in the case of long-term rehabilitation, a "process of resocialization may be necessary through which the incapacitated individual must learn to establish new relationships with those around him" (Suchman, 1965, p. 116). In the case of chronic illness, this stage may present serious medical problems. However, most individuals welcome this stage and return rather easily to former roles.

Segall (1976) reviews 20 years of research on Parsons' concept of the sick role and concludes that "the extent to which this theoretical model contributes to a greater understanding of the way in which the sick person actually thinks, feels and behaves still awaits empirical verification" (p. 168). The Parsonian concept according to Segall, is best illustrated by "temporary, acute physical illness," and evidence suggests that the sick role is affected by social, cultural, and personal factors as well as by the nature of the illness.

The importance of such factors is illustrated by the work of Zola (1966), who interviewed patients of different ethnic groups about their symptoms. Comparisons of Irish and Italian patients showed a pattern of differences in the complaints presented (even when the disorder was the same), with the Irish patients "limiting and understating their difficulties and the Italians spreading and generalizing theirs" (p. 624). Zola attempts to account for these differences in terms of the cultural differences between the two groups. As Zola points out:

> While there has long been recognition of the subjectivity and variability of a patient's reporting of his symptoms, there has been little attention to the fact that this reporting may be influenced by systematic social factors like ethnicity. Awareness of the influence of this and similar factors can be of considerable aid in the practical problems of diagnosis and treatment of many diseases, particularly where the diagnosis is dependent to a large extent on what the patient is able and willing, or thinks important enough, to tell the doctor" (p. 629).

Gordon (1966) demonstrated the importance of socioeconomic status in validating an individual as "sick." There were no differences between socioeconomic groups in terms of behavioral expectancies of the sick person once the definition was made, but differences were found by Gordon in the "conceptions of who is and who is not sick" (p. 99). Gordon's findings support the idea of a "sick role" that is used when the prognosis is serious and uncertain. In cases where the prognosis is known and not serious, the set of behavioral expectations are referred to as the "impaired role," and persons seen as occupying this role are under social pressure by others to maintain normal activities.

In a more recent restatement of his concept of the sick role (1975), Parsons points out that he had never intended to restrict the concept of the sick role to "deviant behavior" or to acute illness. Nor did he mean to imply that the role of the patient is completely passive. Indeed with less acute illness, the active participation of the client may be substantial. However, Parsons contends, the patient-physician relationship is basically an asymmetrical one since "there must be a built-in institutionalized superiority of the professional roles, grounded in responsibility, competence, and occupational concern" (Parsons, 1975, p. 271). He views the relationship between the full-time career professional and the lay person (client) as inherently asymmetrical and hierarchical with respect to issues concerning health and illness, in the same way that there is a built-in asymmetry between professor and student or lawyer and client.

OTHER VIEWS OF THE CLIENT ROLE

A somewhat different view of the client's role is presented by Tagliacozzo and Mauksch (1972) who interviewed hospitalized patients concerning their perceptions of how hospital personnel expected them to act. There was a great deal of consistency in their view of the rules governing being a "good" patient, with the physician seen as expecting "trust and confidence" and "cooperation." Nurses were seen to expect patients to be "cooperative," "respectful," "considerate," and "not to be demanding." Furthermore, these were the characteristics that the patients attempted to project in the interviews. Pointing out that patients see few areas in which they have control and hesitate to deviate from acceptable behavior for fear they will not be given the services needed, the authors speculate that:

> The feeling of helplessness of patients is partly derived from an incapacity to judge adequately the competence of those who take care of them — in part, from the fact that their experiences do not provide easily defendable criteria for asserting their rights, and partly from their reluctance to use the controls which are available to them (p. 172).

The patients knew what was expected of *them*, but were much more unsure of what they should expect of *others*. "The interviews reflect a degree of uncertainty whether physicians and nurses operate as effective teams in close communication or whether the patient ought to function as interpreter and intermediary between these two all important functionaries" (Tagliacozzo and Mauksch, 1972, p. 174). Thus patients' attempts to be "good" patients may be frustrated by the communication problems that may hinder their attempts to control their situation.

Coser (1956) analyzed the role of medical and surgical patients in a general hospital on the basis of standardized interviews of 51 patients at the time of discharge. Coser found two orientations toward hospital life among the patients interviewed. For some patients the hospital was seen as a source of "care and attention" that provided for the gratification of *primary needs*. For other patients the functions of the hospital were seen as *limited* and *instrumental*. These attitudes were also seen in the patient's image of the "good" doctor as either an omnipotent figure who dispenses "protection and love" (meets primary needs) or as the competent professional (instrumental). Patients were found to differ in their attitudes toward the patient role on the basis of whether their orientation to the hospital and the doctor were *primary* or *instrumental*. Primary patients were more likely to see the "good" patient as one who accepted hospital norms and was submissive to hospital demands, while instrumental patients felt the "good" patient should show some autonomy and self-sufficiency. In general, Coser's results suggested that primary patients made a better adjustment to hospital life than did instrumental patients, but that the latter were better prepared to return to their normal lives.

In contrast to the Parsonian version of the sick role, which according to Lorber (1975) is applicable only to outpatients, "inpatient care imposes on patients a role characterized by submission to professional authority, enforced cooperation, and depersonalized status" (p. 214), and patients may comply with expectations in part for fear that they will not be properly taken care of unless they are "good." However, patients may differ in the extent to which they accept the role of the compliant patient.

Lorber examined surgery patients with conforming and deviant attitudes toward the hospital patient role and found those with deviant attitudes were more argumentative and complaining and were more often labeled "problem patients" before they left the hospital. On the other hand, very passive, conforming patients were not always seen as "good" by the staff, since at times they failed to ask for needed attention. In general, Lorber found that "good" patients were those who caused the staff little trouble and did not interfere with hospital routine, while those regarded as "problem" patients were the seriously ill, who demanded a great deal of attention, and the not seriously ill, who complained and were uncooperative. "[The latter] problem patients, in this study, were tranquilized, sometimes discharged early, and, in one case, referred to a psychiatrist — types of response to willful, troublesome patients other researchers have also found" (Lorber, 1975, p. 224).

The physician's view of the patient is described by Ort, Ford, and Liske (1974) who examined sources of satisfaction and dissatisfaction among medical students, faculty, and practitioners. The doctors reported their greatest satisfaction came from "giving help and care," "personal affiliation with patients," and using "legitimate rational control," while their greatest dissatisfaction came from a lack of control, which was mainly attributed to patients. Dissatisfaction was expressed with "patients who are difficult to manage, refractory, demanding, self-centered, uncooperative, or rebellious" (p. 31).

Variations in the doctor-patient relationship were perceived by Szasz and Hollender (1956) who identified the following three models:

1. **Activity-Passivity.** The patient plays a passive role; the physician does something to the patient. Like the parent-infant relationship in some ways, this type of relationship may be appropriate for situations in which the patient is helpless (such as acute emergencies). Here the physician has absolute control and to some extent must "disidentify" with the patient as a person.

2. **Guidance-Cooperation.** The patient is expected to cooperate with (or obey) the physician; the doctor tells the patient what to do. More like the relationship between parent and adolescent, the physician is still in charge and expects all directions to be followed. Both participants are active but the physician has more power.

3. **Mutual Participation.** Patients are helped to help themselves; the physician relates to the patient as to another adult. In some ways the doctor may act as a consultant to patients who carry out much of their own treatment, as with diabetics who administer their own insulin. In diabetes it is essential that patients be active partners in the treatment process. In a situation of mutuality, it is necessary that the parties are of equal power, are interdependent, and that the activities are satisfying to both. The satisfaction in this kind of relationship cannot come from the power or control that the physician exerts over the patient.

As the authors point out, changes in the patient's condition may necessitate changes in the relationship, so that as the patient moves from a crisis state to an acute one and then to a chronic or rehabilitation state, it would be appropriate for the relationship to move in the direction of more active participation on the part of the patient. Warning that some might think one approach better or more "ethical" than another, in particular "that it is better to identify with the patient than to treat him like a helplessly sick person" (Szasz and Hollender, 1956, p. 438), they suggest that each model is appropriate at certain times and inappropriate at others. Changes in the type of relationship require flexibility of both patient and helper. Where both become dissatisfied with each other, "the physician usually feels that the patient is 'uncooperative' and 'difficult,' whereas the patient regards the physician as 'unsympathetic' and lacking in understanding of his unique needs. Both are correct" (pp. 438-439). Such problems with a changing relationship may well lead to a "dissolution" of the relationship, as the patient seeks a new doctor and the doctor in turn moves on to other patients who will benefit from her or his approach.

Finally, Wilson and Bloom (1972) in their review of the patient-practitioner relationship, point out that "the Parsonian assertion that the roles of treater and client must be mutually understood and mutually rewarded does not at all mean that practitioners and patients are equals in the therapeutic situation" (p. 318). They explain further:

> As the skilled person meets the unskilled and tries to alter the latter, the parties can no more be equals than are parent and child or teacher and student. The helping agent, it is asserted, must have leverage to induce change; this leverage is generated by over-all circumstances, notably the *professional prestige* and *situational authority* of the health agent and the *situational dependency* of the patient (p. 318).

The power of practitioners rests in their expertise and their ability to provide what the patient "wants and needs," while the dependency of patients lies in their social and psychological vulnerability as "sick" persons. Social class and cultural differences between patient and helper will only exacerbate the barriers in communication and heighten the problems in the patient-professional relationship.

THE CLIENT AND THE TEAM APPROACH

The models of the client role and the client-professional relationship examined in this chapter focus on the traditional dyadic relationship between the "sick" person and an individual who attempts to help. Although this has been the most common pattern of medical services and has generally served as a model for other professionals in their relationships with clients, there are a variety of service delivery systems available today that reflect different models of the client-professional relationship. This includes, of course, the team approach.

According to Wilson (1970),

> The most pronounced shift in the traditional Western therapeutic dyad is probably a departure from the dyad itself. Increasingly, the patient is involved not in an isolated two-person social system but in a medical team effort in which the physician is first among equals rather than unique healer. A paramount issue of the future may be the redefinition of the doctor's role as a collaborative one and the patterning of team medicine for maximum therapeutic efficacy. The future of medical practice will probably rest on a detailed meshing of medicine, nursing, social work, administration, and perhaps even social science (p. 31).

What kinds of changes in the relationship between client and professional result from the team approach? We can see a number of possible effects. First, it might be expected that as Wilson (1970) indicated, the degree of dependency in the relationship between client and professional cannot be as great when a number of health agents are involved. Thus, although *more* professionals are involved, and consequently clients may have a better chance of finding one with whom they can develop a comfortable relationship, the strength of each of those relationships is likely to be less intense than if only one team member were clearly involved with the client. This dilution of the relationship affects both patient and professional. While the patient whose welfare rests on a number of professional workers may feel less dependent on any one of them, the professional may at the same time experience less personal responsibility for the client and perhaps even feel a diminished sense of accomplishment when treatment is successfully completed.

Second, clients' lessened dependency on any one member of the team and the fact that at times they may receive contradictory information from various team members suggests that the treatment process might become more confusing for some team-treated clients. Illness and hospitalization generally produce heightened anxiety and a sense of helplessness in the client, and the client may feel an increased need for structure and for clear communication. If the patient is unsure which team member can be asked to supply clarification and additional information, the team situation could create more problems for the patient.

Third, members of the team, particularly if it is a strong, cohesive working group, may find that their primary job satisfaction has shifted from working with clients to working with other team members. Since goals for the client have now become team goals, reaching those goals may no longer give the same sense of personal reward, but are now important in terms of the *team's* accomplishment. The team may actually become more important to the professional than the client.

Fourth, clients may be given more responsibility for their own care and be expected to play a more active role than in the past. Clients may more often be included as active participants in team conferences and asked to play a major role in decision making and treatment planning.

Fifth, the family is also more likely to be included in the planning process if a team is involved. Since a number of specialists are concerned with all aspects of the client's functioning, inclusion of appropriate family members seems a natural step.

Finally, the overall quality of care received by the client may well be better with a team approach than with a traditional dyadic relationship. Both the treatment of existing conditions and the prevention of potential problems may be more effective under an interdisciplinary team, thus enhancing the client-professional relationship.

While many clients will welcome such changes, some may find them disturbing. For example, the patients identified by Coser (1956) as *primary* (i.e., those who expect to have primary needs taken care of by the hospital) may not welcome the more active role implied by the team concept. Such patients tend to look upon the doctor as omnipotent and seem to find that reassuring. On the other hand, Coser's *instrumental* patients view the "good" patient as one who is relatively autonomous and self-sufficient rather than submissive and compliant.

The view of the client as an active participant in treatment is not a new one. Not all professionals have adopted the hierarchical, asymmetrical dyad as a model of client-professional interaction. Psychotherapists and counselors have traditionally tended to emphasize the need to develop a therapeutic relationship in which the client assumes a major responsibility for treatment and plays an active role. Most striking in the "nondirective" or "client-centered" approach of Carl Rogers (1951), this view is held to some extent by most proponents of psychotherapy. The increasing popularity of family therapy and group therapy reflects further departures from the asymmetrical dyad.

The idea that clients may serve as comanagers in their own rehabilitation has been discussed by Wright (1960). "The principle of comanagement is an apt designation for the kind of relationship advocated. It connotes active participation by *both* client and specialist" (p. 345). Such a relationship enhances the client's self-respect and increases motivation. Furthermore, according to Wright, the counselor often does not have sufficient knowledge to make important decisions affecting the client's future, and some decisions may well fall within the "inalienable rights" of the client to self-determination.

More recently, legislation has specified the participation of clients and family members in treatment and educational planning. For example, Individualized Written Rehabilitation Programs require the signature of the client receiving services from the state-federal rehabilitation programs. Similarly, Public Law 94-142 requires parental approval of a child's Individualized Educational Program (IEP) if the child is receiving special education services, and provides for due process hearings if the parents do not support the decisions reached.

For the team member, the changing role of the client may be a mixed blessing. While many professionals welcome a more active role for their clients, the client's participation in team meetings sometimes calls for adjustments that may be difficult for some members. When clients become members of the team, team interactions may become more inhibited, communication may become more formal, and reports may be considerably abbreviated. In extreme cases the team conference may become a mere formality, with the real decisions made outside the team meeting. Sometimes the addition of clients to the team can be seen as primarily a political move designed to shift the balance of power in the team, "open up" the decision process, or respond to consumer pressure.

Finally, it should be reemphasized that whatever the role of a particular client vis-à-vis the professionals on the team, the client remains the major focus of the team's efforts. The problems presented by the client define what the team is to do and who is to do it. If the client is dependent on the team for treatment and care, the team is equally dependent on the client for its continued functioning. The client *is* the reason for the existence of the team.

Chapter 5

Organizational Settings

The professionals who constitute an interdisciplinary team are generally members of some human service organization such as a hospital, school, community mental health center, or rehabilitation agency. This chapter explores the impact of the organizational setting on the functioning of the team.

In one sense, the "parent" organization defines the team, its members, its tasks, and to some extent the place and time of its interaction. Thus how the team operates is markedly influenced by its organizational setting. Some of the characteristics of an organization that will influence the functioning of the team are the type of organization and its goals, the structure, the locus of authority and control, and the organization's norms and values. Such characteristics are influential no matter what type of human service institution is involved.

TYPES OF ORGANIZATIONS

Human service institutions may be classified by means of the source of control (i.e., governmental or nongovernmental) or by function (i.e., medical care, teaching, or other activities).

Governmental organizations include a variety of facilities and agencies at the city, county, state, and federal levels. Federal agencies include military, veterans, and public health organizations, while nonfederal agencies include institutions controlled at other governmental levels such as state schools and hospitals. In some cases, control might be shared, as when federal grants support state- or locally-directed projects and federal guidelines exert some control over the programs. Nongovernmental institutions include voluntary (or nonprofit) as well as proprietary (or profit-making) agencies.

Health care institutions include hospitals, extended care facilities, and other institutions offering inpatient services, as well as clinics and other outpatient institutions and agencies providing home care. In addition there are a large number of health-related institutions including schools and social service and welfare agencies.

The type of institution in which the team operates can be a major factor in determining the clientele served, what programs are offered, and the staff people hired (Coe, 1970). In these and other ways, the type of institution has a significant impact on the type of team that operates within its walls and the way that team is structured and functions.

While there has been a great deal written concerning the place of organizational theory and organizational development in human service institutions, it would seem that as yet there is no entirely adequate basis for organizational analysis and development in what Drucker termed the 'Third Sector' (i.e., service organizations). Indeed, Drucker (1978) in regard to such organizations says:

> Both the businessman and the civil servant tend to underrate the difficulty of managing service institutions. The businessman thinks it's all a matter of being efficient, the civil servant thinks it's all a matter of having the right procedures and controls. Both are wrong — service institutions are more complex than either businesses or government agencies — as we are painfully finding out in our attempts to make the hospital a little more manageable (no one to my knowledge has yet tried to do this with the university).
>
> Indeed we know far too little about managing the service institution — it is simply too recent a phenomenon. But we do know that it needs to be managed. And we do know that defining what its task is and what it should not be is the most essential step in making the service institutions of the Third Sector manageable, managed and performing.

It is, however, possible to look at some of the characteristics of human service organizations and see how they may relate to team functioning. In doing so it must be remembered that the dominant organizational pattern in Western society is _bureaucratic_. The bureaucratic organization is hierarchical, with power and authority concentrated at higher levels in the organization. As Kingdon (1973) puts it:

> formal rules and scalar authority, or hierarchy, bear the main burden of socially integrating our organizations and mobilizing our resources . . . individuals in our organization relinquish their power to the scalar authority of officials who are then charged with the responsibility for establishing formal rules controlling resource allocation and socially integrating the organization (pp. 1-2).

In addition to a hierarchical authority structure undergirded by a system of rules and procedures, bureaucratic organizations generally are characterized by a differentiation of tasks performed by individuals and by subunits of the organization.

The fact is, the ways in which human service institutions are organized have a major influence on the operation of the team. All human service organizations have a number of attributes in common, all of which have some impact on the interdisciplinary team.

The organization *exists in a social context* and interacts with that context in both a proactive and reactive manner. It is therefore an open system receiving input from the environment and in turn generating some form of output. Development of the organization is based on some *identified human need.* Such needs may change over a period of time. Indeed, the organization that does not undergo modification in accord with changing human needs will cease to exist. Most often, organizations do modify their activities to address changing needs, although this change may lag well behind the identification of new needs.

The organization is based on some *belief* or *theory* of the nature of man, the nature of society, or nature of the universe; it may also be based on a specific theory that conditions its structure, goals, and activities. *Resources* and *energy* are utilized by organizations to produce some *believed social good.*

To accomplish that social good, organizations will adopt, utilize, or exhibit some of the following characteristics: explicit or implicit goals and objectives, patterns of authority and decision making, communication, rewards and sanctions, norms and values. They are composed of and address specific populations with roles and membership within the organization. They occupy space. They employ various processes and technologies in achieving their outcomes.

Goals and Objectives

When goals are set by a superordinate authority, they may differ from the goals of any one team member or the team as a whole. For example, when case loads are set at higher levels than the team considers consistent with adequate client care, the team goals of "effective" client care are in conflict with a goal of "efficient" care on the part of an authority structure.

Perrow (1961) discusses two kinds of goals in a complex organization. First are the *official goals* which are:

> general purposes of the organization as put forth in the charter, annual reports, public statements by key executives and other authoritative pronouncements. . . . The official goal of a hospital may be to promote the health of the community through curing the ill, and sometimes through preventing illness, teaching and conducting research (p. 855).

Such goals are often deliberately vague and abstract, and in order to adequately understand organizational behavior it is necessary to examine a second type of goal — what Perrow calls *operative goals*. As the name suggests, operative goals refer to the operating policies of the organization; "they tell us what the organization actually is trying to do, regardless of what the official goals say are the aims" (p. 855).

Even when operative goals are quite clear, it does not necessarily mean that the goals of the team or of any team member will coincide with the goals of the parent organization. For example, Banta and Fox (1972), in their study of a health care team in a poverty community found that:

> Everyone on the professional staff with the exception of the "Public Health" physicians was dedicated to giving comprehensive, high quality, family-oriented medical care to the poor people of Columbia Point. The "Public Health" physicians fundamentally disagreed with this goal: one such physician states "the rationale behind Columbia Point — the premise — complete comprehensive care for the poor is good; they've got no care. I'm not sure they're warranted to as good care as some one who can afford more. . . . If they can't pay, it's a shame, and if we were a society with medical care distributed evenly, it would be good, but it isn't. But . . . as to the basic premise, that I agree with, that someone who pays more gets more" (p. 702).

It may be seen that when the goals of the team or of some team members differ significantly from those of the organization, there may be a negative impact on the functioning of the team. Similarly, when the team as a whole questions the organizational goals, team functions in terms of those goals may be greatly impaired. As a result the team disintegrates or begins to develop its own set of goals that may be at variance with those of the parent organization.

Authority and Decision Making

The locus of authority may condition how the team functions since the authority structure does indeed determine the overall goals of the organization and how those goals are to be achieved. Let us take as a case in point the development of the general hospital as an agency typical of those providing human services to a range of clients.

"The large general hospital is the prototype of the multi-purpose organization; it is a hotel and a school, a laboratory and a stage for treatment" (Wilson, 1963). This, of course, has not always been so. Before medical science began its accelerated progress early in this century, hospitals tended to be places of refuge for the homeless and the poor, who had no one else to care for them. In view of the high death rates in such settings, only those who had no other place to go consented to hospitalization. Thus it was not until medical treatment markedly improved and hospital insurance was readily available that a large portion of the population came to accept the hospital as a place of treatment (Wilson, 1963, 1970).

During this time of growth and change, the goals of the organization shifted from primarily altruistic and religious aims to the typical goals of the modern hospital — treatment of patients, medical research, and training of health care personnel. However, as with any large, complex, multipurpose organization, there is always the possibility for conflict and divisiveness over priorities and the use of resources. As the power base shifts among various individuals and groups within the organization, there may well be accompanying shifts in goals. How this has occurred during the emergence of the modern hospital has been delineated by Perrow (1961, 1963).

Perrow discusses the four different types of authority structures that have emerged as hospitals developed and how these structures have shaped the operative goals of the institution.

1. **Trustee domination.** In hospitals dominated by their board of trustees, the emphasis is likely to be on capital investments and community acceptance of the hospital, and the operative goals tend to focus on the "role of trustees as community representatives and contributors to community health" (p. 858). In the early years of the modern hospital when actual treatment was rare and activities were focused on caring for the *poor* sick, rather than for those who could afford care, community acceptance was a major goal, and hospital trustees tended to be extremely powerful. The basis of their control is generally financial, and when they choose to wield their power they may control everything from hiring and promotion to "the brand of grape juice" ordered.

2. **Medical domination.** The source of power for physicians lies in their professional knowledge and skills. Technical competence gives control over new technological resources, and as these increased historically, so did the power of the doctor. Although as Wilson (1963) has noted, the medical staff are often characterized as "guests" in the hospital, in fact they operate as a kind of "shadow" organization and are in an excellent position to gain control. Operative goals in such a setting tend for the most part to be medical — the physicians may see the hospital primarily as a place to bring their private patients.

3. **Administrative dominance.** Dominance by hospital administrators is based "first, on the need for coordinating the increasingly complex, nonroutinizable functions hospitals have undertaken . . . a second, related basis for control stems from the fact that health services in general have become increasingly interdependent and specialized" (Perrow, 1961, p. 859). As hospitals became more complex institutions involved in a complicated network of interrelated facilities, the training, experience, and time available to administrators better equipped them to deal with internal affairs as well as with relationships with other

agencies and hospitals. An administrator's dominance may lead toward operative goals with an emphasis on efficiency and budget control.

4. **Multiple leadership.** When no one group is dominant enough to control the others, there is multiple leadership, "a division of labor regarding the determination of goals and the power to achieve them" (p. 861). This pattern of leadership is likely to occur in organizations with multiple goals "which lack precise criteria of achievement and admit of considerable tolerance with regard to achievement (p. 861). One can easily discern how different power sources might view the operation of the interdisciplinary team in different ways, thereby affecting its performance.

The shift in patterns of power in the hospital has been described by Wilson (1959) who notes the change in the role of the hospital physician from unchallenged master to bureaucratic functionary. This role change is due partly to the increased specialization of the physician, the growing complexity of the hospital, and the professionalization of the hospital administrator and auxiliary health care workers. The parallel chains of medical authority and administrative authority overlap and produce confusion. Wilson cites a case study of *Aprilton,* a relatively small, semirural hospital that was reorganized when a professional hospital administrator was brought in by the trustees to deal with twin problems of physical deterioration and decreasing quality of care. With the support of the trustees (and an increased exercise of power on their part), the administrator was able to make a necessary reorganization of the medical staff. The measure of the change was the significantly better rating given the hospital by the American College of Surgeons — from 45 percent adequacy to 77 percent just four years later.

In discussing the changing role of the doctor, Wilson comments on the change from the old independent "charismatic" role in the doctor-dominated hospital to the new role of the physician as *team member*.

As team member the doctor in the hospital finds his performance conditioned by interaction with a number of allied specialists . . . with non physicians (nurse, social worker, medical librarian, administrator) as well as with those specialists whose medical competencies adjoin his own (pathologist, radiologist, etc.). He confronts a matrix of collaboration which he cannot expect to dominate or hope to avoid.

The doctor in a team has even been viewed by some as a professional who is suffering from a drastic loss of function. Not only has the physician necessarily adopted a more limited and less authoritative role, such observers maintain, but he has been in many instances reduced to a kind of ceremonious middle man whose chief work is to mediate between the patient and an array of technical and specialized resources for both diagnosis and treatment (Wilson, 1959, p. 182).

Thus we see how one of the major providers of client services, the general hospital, has moved through a series of power shifts as it moved toward bureaucratization. Other organizations have experienced similar shifts in power as new professions and new specialists have emerged to challenge the existing systems. These inherent conflicts between various power centers must be understood and resolved if we hope to provide coordinated care to the clients served in these organizational settings.

Today many vestiges of the doctor-dominated system are evident and are likely to remain. However, the professionalization of other health personnel (including the administrator) offers some balance to the power of the physician. There are changes in the agency governing board as "community representative" comes to mean housewife and laborer as well as business leader and professional, and this also leads to shifts in the goals and priorities of the organization. It should be kept in mind that the hospital and other service agencies are not the independent monoliths they sometimes appear to be. They are, in fact, highly dependent on support from the society in which they operate, and their existence must continually be justified, not only to the community but to a number of federal, state, and local regulatory bodies and professional organizations.

The rising consumer movement in health care has tended to focus on two demands made on hospitals and other agencies: community representation on governing boards and availability of services to the surrounding community (Croog and Ver Steeg, 1972; Johnson, 1970). These demands run counter to the traditional professional view that the patient lacks knowledge concerning health care and related issues. One source of professional power has always been *unique* expertise — this is the basis for society's willingness to confer such autonomy on the professional. The consumer movement strongly threatens that autonomy; it is no longer assumed that the patient is incapable of evaluating the services rendered by the health care facility and the professional. These issues are sometimes fought out at meetings of the board of trustees or at open meetings of the citizens advisory council. In some cases such councils have acquired veto power over major appointments within the agency. As consumers come to play an increasingly important role as advisers to various service organizations (including regulatory bodies and licensing boards), the conflict between professional and consumer priorities can be expected to cause real difficulties.

Concurrent with these changes, there has been an increase in community involvement through governmental bodies at various levels, as illustrated by the case of one hospital that was required to submit 105 reports and/or inspections in one year to various governmental agencies (Croog and Ver Steeg, 1972; Pomrinse, 1969). Another external force with which the hospital must deal are the various health insurance organizations involved in third party payment for services rendered in and by the hospital. Such organizations can withhold appropriate reimbursement if the hospital fails to make certain internal changes. In short, these groups can wield considerable influence over actual procedures used by the professional and by the human service agency.

Thus control of an organization is likely to be a complex compromise of internal and external forces characterized by a multitude of conflicting values, goals, and priorities. As the power structure shifts in response to changing pressures within the agency and outside it, the goals and priorities will also shift, with corresponding changes in "what people do" within the agency.

Lines of Communication

As the knowledge base of human service organizations has expanded, there has been an increased need for additional types of professionals — and consequently an increase in the division of labor and degree of specialization. In bureaucratic organizations this has been equated with more efficient use of manpower. But such specialization has in many instances led to such fragmented care that no one is really taking care of the client as a total person. The development of the team approach may indeed be a direct response to this situation.

The division of labor and separation of function within the organization has brought concomitant problems in communication. Most organizations are set up in a way that is in natural conflict with the team approach. There seems to be an almost slavish adherence to the notion that individuals with similar functions should be housed and administered as units. Among the factors that tend to reinforce such a structure are the need to identify with a particular professional group who speak the same language, an unfamiliarity with the other professions, and the need to house certain types of equipment together (e.g., X-ray, laboratories, physical therapy equipment, etc.).

The communication system also tends to reinforce the development of units along professional lines. For example, the organizational chart for a general hospital typically shows each service (e.g., nursing, social work, occupational therapy) as a separate unit reporting to the administrator of the hospital. A similar situation can be found in many large human service organizations such as schools and rehabilitation centers where the psychologist reports to the chief of psychology, the special educator to the head of that division, the regular teacher to a supervisor, and so forth. We shall ignore for the time being the dual nature of authority in many health service organizations since this introduces still another degree of complexity. What is immediately apparent is that under this system use of the team approach may lead to some confusion in lines of communication and authority.

When each professional is responsible both to a team and to a functional unit, there is the distinct possibility that there may be divided and therefore, in some cases, ineffective leadership and authority. This has the effect of blurring lines of communication and increasing the possibility of confusion and conflict. The result is reduced efficiency in client services. As Beckhard (1974) quotes from the director of the Martin Luther King, Jr. Health Center:

> We are having a lot of difficulties in the operation of the health teams.
> . . . [Some of the difficulties center around] information flow and record
> keeping. Patient records are often incomplete and in the wrong place at
> the wrong time. A number of referrals get lost between departments and
> between the center and the hospital. . . . Each functional department
> head . . . has his functional counterparts on the delivery team reporting
> to him and tends naturally to be more concerned with his own functional
> area than with the overall management of the center (p. 70).

Thus we can see the crux of this particular problem: the team consists of individuals who believe they owe their primary allegiance and responsibility to a functionally organized unit or department, while the secondary group (i.e., the team) only provides a convenient battleground upon which interprofessional and interdepartmental wars are fought. In a dispute between a "team leader" and a department head, it is not difficult to see where the individual professional will probably stand, particularly if decisions about promotions and salary rest with the departmental unit.

Processes

Large organizations in general attempt to rationalize their operations by adopting standard procedures. These are the rules by which the institution deals both with its clientele and with its internal operations. Over a period of time these rules tend to become solidified and are codified into procedure manuals and similar publications. Unfortunately such systems of rules are seldom client-centered, but instead tend to focus on the organization and its internal needs. Since most human service organizations are organized on disciplinary lines of authority, rules tend to be written in this way, with consequent reinforcement of the existing structure.

An example of the abrogation of team responsibility to procedural considerations is reported in a slightly tongue-in-cheek manner by Hirschowitz (1973):

> *The Superintendent's Discharge Conference.* This conference
> dramatizes one of the many paradoxes inherent in the psychiatric institu-
> tion's decision making: the person who makes the significant decision is
> furthest removed from the patient, has the least data about him, and has
> observed him in the fewest interactional contexts. On the other hand,
> those who do know the patient and are best able to predict his behavior
> wield least influence in deciding what is best for him.
>
> The Superintendent's Discharge Conference is patterned on a judicial
> model (not unmixed with Kafkaesque ingredients). A summary is pre-

sented of the patient's admission status, subsequent course, and present status; team members read evidence; then a patient advocate, usually his physician, pleads the discharge case for his patient-client. The superintendent functions in the dual role of judge and prosecutor (society's advocate). In this role he hears the evidence, interviews the client, then pronounces judgment. More often than not, the decision is responsive to the presumed expectations of the community, particularly the original dispatchers or complainants (p. 52).

Thus we can see that the procedures of an institution may not, in effect, reinforce team efforts.

Rewards, Sanctions, Norms, and Values

The manner in which the individual is held accountable to the organization influences behavior. In bureaucratic organizations, rewards and sanctions are applied in terms that are not always consonant with the avowed goals of the organization. For example, in universities there is much said about the virtues of excellent teaching, but promotions are based for the most part on research and publication. Similarly, if the organization mouths pious platitudes about the virtue of working in teams, but bases its actual reward structure on the individual achievement within a disciplinary context, teamwork may be much less valued.

Support for this contention is found in the study by Geigle-Bentz, who concludes that the "opinions of interdisciplinary health care team members toward the team approach, communication, democracy, leadership roles are not consistent with those suggested in the health care literature [concerning teams]" (Geigle-Bentz, 1975, p. 118). In other words, in a study of what team members actually thought about the team approach, it was found that their opinions varied markedly from those normally found in what people write about teams.

The reward structure may be such that teamwork goes relatively unnoticed. If promotions, pay raises, and similar extrinsic rewards are based on recognition by disciplinary units of the organization, most staffers will make their greatest efforts in these areas. In addition to the extrinsic reward system there may also exist an intrinsic system that ties in with departmental disciplinary organization rather than with the team structure. Such systems often are reinforced by their congruence with the values and norms of the various professions.

Membership and Roles

The organization defines who will be a member of a team and what role that individual will play on the team. Definitions may be informal or very highly structured, with written descriptions of the job and the necessary qualifications for membership. Since these descriptions are generally written in terms of the formal or operative goals of the organization, they may not accurately reflect the roles actually played by the various team members or the team as a whole. For example, in writing about rehabilitation teams, Horwitz says:

> A professional role may be nicely defined in a formal agency job description explicitly indicating prescribed and optional activities, implicitly suggesting that there are certain tasks more appropriately performed by workers in some other job title. But in the crucible of practice, performance will vary from the "ideal type" because of individual differences in understanding of role and reciprocal role-limited behavior of colleagues. Also, as a result of individual differences of skill in role performance and in overall effectiveness — that is in problem solving activities — a variety of professionally appropriate orientations to the job is to be expected. (Horwitz, 1969, p. 38).

It is readily seen that individual and/or team orientations to professional roles may be in conflict with bureaucratically prescribed functions. Such conflict may lead to attendant problems in defining team functions and subsequent loss of team and organizational effectiveness. If, indeed, one of the characteristics of a profession is autonomous action and self-regulation, this is at odds with bureaucratic organizational structure.

Spatial Relationships

Physical location is an important aspect of how the organization influences team functioning. If for example a team were housed in one office with adjoining desks, it is more likely that informal interaction would take place than if team members were housed in separate offices in different wings of the building. Similarly, the spatial arrangements for conferences and other meetings can have great bearing on how the team members interact.

INTERORGANIZATIONAL RELATIONSHIPS

In addition to the influence of *intra*organizational characteristics on the team, forces generated by *inter*organizational relationships also have impact on team functioning.

The relationships *between* organizations has been examined by Levine and White (1972). Although interorganizational relationships continue to grow in complexity since their study was conducted, many of their findings and interpretations seem relevant to other settings and other times. They investigated the interaction of 22 health organizations in a medium-sized New England community. Included in the 22 agencies were 5 hospitals, 3 governmental organizations (health, welfare, and school), and 14 voluntary agencies. Since no agency has unlimited resources, health organizations usually limit their functions to those they can expertly handle. This being the case, most agencies find it is necessary to exchange resources or elements with other organizations. "The need for a sufficient number of clients, for example, is often more efficiently met through exchange with other organizations than through independent case finding procedures" (Levine and White, 1972, p. 587).

The researchers identify three main types of elements exchanged between health agencies: referral of clients; services of professionals, volunteers and other personnel; and other resources including equipment, funds, and information. Thus patients may be sent from one agency to another for additional services; a professional from the second agency may provide these services and the first agency will pay the second for these services. It was found that interorganizational exchange was determined by the functions of the interacting organizations as well as by prestige, leadership, and other factors.

Exchange, however, is only one factor in interorganizational relationships. Competition for scarce resources, whether from public or private sources, often affects the way in which institutions interrelate. Such competitive situations often discourage teamwork when members of the team are from different organizations. For example, one institution's need for numbers of patients to fill beds may reduce the chances that a client will be transferred to another institution where more adequate care might be given.

THE BUREAUCRATIC MODEL

Throughout this chapter, we have examined the impact of bureaucratic organization on the team. It is apparent that the adaptation of the bureaucratic model to the human service sector has not been as successful as it was in the early stages of industrialization in the business sector. The worker-organization relationship does not seem to be the same in industry and in human service institutions. In fact, continued attempts to impose more bureaucratic structures on human service organizations often lead to frustration and dysfunction in terms of client service.

A number of authors including Drucker (1978) and Wiesbord (1976) have pointed to the differences between the industrial model of organization and that of the human service field. One obvious source of conflict comes from the interaction of the professional and the organization. Taken at its simplest level, the professional is by definition autonomous, while organizations have as their main function the "direction and control of human behavior." Organizations are largely predicated on the idea that rational division of tasks is an appropriate way to maximize the delivery of services. In practice, the professional in the human service organization may function as a caregiver one moment, as a teacher or student the next moment, and as a researcher during the next. The tasks are complex and at times defy rational division. Indeed the development of the team approach may have been in large part due to an inappropriate application of the principle of division of tasks. Fragmentation of care has often resulted to the detriment of the client.

"Matrix organization" attempts to deal with the conflict between bureaucratic organizations and the team approach by setting up a dual organizational pattern or matrix. Each individual has a position in the matrix that permits communication on both a horizontal and vertical basis. Tichy (1977) provides an excellent case study of the development of a matrix organization in a primary care setting. Tichy outlines the development of the matrix organization at the Dr. Martin Luther King Jr. Health Center and points to the opportunities and difficulties of operating in a setting that contains a dual reporting and authority system. For such a system to work, all levels of the organization must be prepared to deal openly and creatively with conflict or with emphasis of one axis of the matrix over another.

It would seem that Drucker is right: we do not know enough about the human service institution. Neither do we know enough about teams and how they function within various types of organizations.

Chapter 6

Team Goals and Activities

If we look at how health care and human service teams spend their time and energy, we find a remarkable diversity of activities. The team approach does not mean that the team members must abandon those activities that define their professional identity. Although there may well be some shifts in the boundaries of professional roles and responsibilities, team members continue to perform many or most of their typical tasks. What is noteworthy about the team concept is the coordination among members of the team, in contrast to the semi-independent stance of more traditional professional roles. Of course, even in nonteam professional interaction, there is necessarily *some* coordination of activities; what is unique about team functioning is the *degree* of such coordination. Team members will still spend considerable time in those activities regarded as their "own territory," but a significant proportion of their time will be used in coordination activities — sharing information about the client's progress and coordinating treatment plans. This kind of coordination is crucial to effective team functioning.

In previous chapters we have examined in some detail the major components of a human service team: the professionals who make up the team, the client to be served, and the organizational setting in which the team operates. Each component brings together a number of variables that may affect the team's behavior directly or indirectly. We are now ready to examine the processes that emerge from the interaction of these components. We will be looking at the next two elements of the Team System Diagram (see Figure 1-1, Chapter One): team goals and activities. We will address questions such as "What is teamwork?", "How do teams interact?", and "What do team members *do*?" In this and the following chapter, the focus will be on team goals and activities undertaken to meet those goals.

TEAM GOALS

Team goals may be regarded as the aims that give direction to the team's actions. Generally goals are agreed on either formally or informally by the majority of team members. Team goals are usually stated in terms of what the team members wish of the team. For example, a health care team in a comprehensive care clinic may state that their primary goal is "to provide effective comprehensive care to residents of this community." General statements of this sort are often supplemented by a number of more specific subgoals related to the diagnosis and treatment of patients, work with families, and patient education.

Teams vary greatly in the extent to which team goals are clearly spelled out and in the number of goals identified. Sometimes team goals are too general and ambiguous to give a clear indication of where the team is heading or what its tasks are. Goals should be stated specifically enough to give direction to the team's activities.

When a team is formed, its principal goal may be articulated either by potential team members or by some external agent that initiates its formation. In either case, considerable effort must be spent in identifying and clarifying these aims, since if the team is to operate as a functioning unit, there must be some sense of shared goals. This does not mean that all members of the team will necessarily "buy into" all of the team goals, or that some participants may not have other goals that have not been agreed upon or even discussed by the group. Such "hidden agenda," although often unarticulated, may be a powerful force serving either to facilitate or disrupt team functioning. Furthermore, a team member's sense of congruence between personal goals and team goals may be an important determinant in his or her enthusiasm and level of participation. A team whose members are unable to articulate and agree upon some minimum number of shared goals is not likely to function effectively for any length of time.

Determinants of Team Goals

When we think of team goals, we tend to think in terms of the team's overall purpose of providing quality services to a client or clients. Certainly client goals are a major portion of the team goals. However, as shown in the Team System Diagram, the three elements we have discussed — professions, organizational context, and the client — all feed into goals that determine team activities.

1. **Client Goals.** The client enters the system with certain goals in mind, such as "I want my symptoms to go away so that I can go back to work," or "I want to receive training so that I can get a job." Part of the task of the team is to help the client meet these goals or in some cases reach more realistic and appropriate goals.

Sometimes the client's family is also involved in setting goals. Child guidance clinics often ask the parent to help set treatment goals, and the IEP team is required to involve parents in determining educational goals for children receiving special education services.

2. **Professional Goals.** Professionals on the team obviously play a crucial role in determining team goals. Some of these goals may seem to be unrelated to the welfare of the client. For example, team members may wish "to increase the status of social work in the hospital," or "to educate other members of the team in the appropriate use of psychological services." Nurses may wish to move toward greater autonomy in their relationships with physicians; occupational therapists may want to clarify professional roles and reduce the extent of role overlap with physical therapy; the special education teacher may wish to provide more consultation to the regular classroom teacher. Whether these professional goals become team goals depends on the extent to which they are understood and accepted by other team members. Unless these goals are clearly articulated, they may remain part of the unverbalized hidden agenda of the individual professional.

3. **Organizational Goals.** Finally, the organization itself contributes to the goals of the team. For example, "to provide quality health care in a cost-effective manner" may be an important goal of the organization that will affect the team goals. Again, whether organizational goals are ever adopted as team goals depends on how well they are communicated to members of the team and accepted by them.

Although the team may not accept all of the goals of the organization, the professionals, or the client, each component will have some measure of influence. The team may express goals such as "adopting a new record-keeping system which will be used on an organization-wide basis," or "utilizing case conferences as teaching sessions to improve professional competence." Although such goals do not deal directly with a specific client, they may ultimately improve the quality of care provided to *all* clients.

Short-Term and Long-Term Goals

Another distinction can be drawn between team goals that are *short-term* (to be accomplished in a minimum period of time) and *long-range* (goals that may take months or even years to reach). Whether the team focuses primarily on short-term or long-term goals depends on the organization in which it functions and how its role is defined. The primary goals for a crisis intervention team, an emergency team, or a surgical team are usually short-term: the major task of the team is to deal with an immediate crisis. Long-term goals are also important to these teams, but immediate priority is given to short-term problems.

In other teams the highest priority is given to long-range problems. For instance, a rehabilitation team working with spinal cord injured patients or a team working with mentally retarded children may focus on goals that are months or even years away. Immediate problems will be handled as they arise, but in such teams the emphasis is on "Where will this client be in one year — or two years — or even five years?" Of course, the team needs to determine intermediate steps in reaching such long-term goals.

For many teams short-term and long-term goals are equally important, and team members engage in a number of activities related to both. In fact, such a balance of goals can be important in the effective functioning of the team. The team that seldom looks at more long-range goals (either for clients or for the team itself) may be avoiding certain issues that present potential conflicts or may have lost a sense of perspective concerning its overall direction. On the other hand, the team that tends to focus only on long-range issues and neglects to develop short-term goals may be avoiding recognition of certain immediate problems.

Task and Maintenance Goals

Most of the goals we have mentioned have involved some task to be completed by the team. This is because teams are primarily task-oriented. This is one of the ways in which human service teams are different from other kinds of groups. However, in addition to these *task-related goals*, the team will also have goals related to the smooth functioning of the group, improving communication among team members, and reducing excessive hostility among members of the team. Such goals are often not clearly recognized or discussed by the human service team, and at times the failure to deal openly with such goals can cause problems in team interaction.

Goals that focus on the group process itself, rather than on team tasks, can be referred to as group maintenance or *team maintenance goals*. Maintenance goals focus on factors that might interfere with the harmony and smooth functioning of the team.

DIMENSIONS OF TEAM GOALS

The relationships among these three dimensions of team goals — *determinant* (client, organization, and professional), *type* (task-related and team-maintenance), and *time* (short-term and long-term) — are illustrated in Figure 6-1. Since the activities of the team follow directly from its goals, the same three dimensions can also be applied to team activities. Some examples of long-term and short-term goals given by the members of a newly formed team may help illustrate the diagram.

- *Short-term task goal:* "to work out a plan of action between now and the time for patient flow to begin"
- *Long-term task goal:* "to demonstrate the treatment of patients in the facility"
- *Short-term team-maintenance goal:* "to learn as much as possible about each team member and her or his expertise"
- *Long-term team maintenance goal:* "to continue clarification of decision-making power: who, what, when, where, and how"

Of the 27 goals on which this team reached consensus, 14 were task-related and 13 were related to team maintenance. The surprisingly large number of team-maintenance goals was probably due to the newness of the team and to some possible ambiguity as to its organizational status. For the same reason there was an emphasis on goals dealing with the organization and with professional roles and relatively little attention given to client-centered goals. In contrast, an ongoing

Figure 6-1 Team Goals and Activities

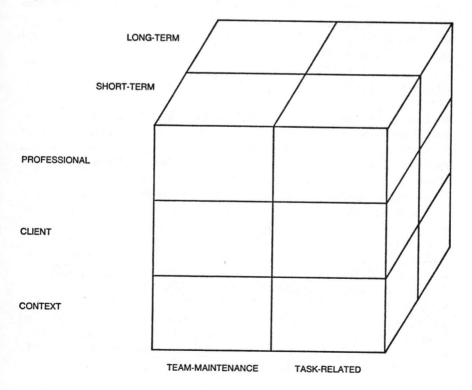

team that has been working together for some time could be expected to have a greater proportion of task-related, client-centered goals.

Goal Conflict

While teams are expected to spend some time initially trying to clarify goals, often there is little attention given to goals once the team has begun to operate because of time pressures and the demand of more immediate tasks. However, when difficulties arise in team functioning, they can often be traced to ambiguous or conflicting goals among team members. For example, the social worker in an outpatient clinic may think that involving the family as participants in the decision-making process is an important team goal. However, if this goal is not shared by other team members, they may resent attempts to involve the family in team meetings.

There are many sources of potential goal conflicts in the team approach. Conflicts may emerge between team members, between the team and the organization, or between team members and the client. Occasional assessment of the team members' perceptions of team goals may prevent some of these problems. Thus an important aspect of team maintenance is the periodic review of team goals, with an attempt to reach or maintain consensus among team members regarding those goals. In Chapter Ten we will explore more fully the concept of goal conflict and how such conflict may be resolved.

TEAM ACTIVITIES

Team goals reflect what it is the team wishes to accomplish. Team activities refer to the actions team members take to reach those goals. Thus team activities can be described along the same dimensions referred to in Figure 6-1. Activities can be task-related or related to team maintenance, short-term or long-term, and focused on the client or the organization or the professional.

The overriding goal of most teams is to attend to the problems presented by a client and produce a specific outcome favorable to that client. The solution to the client's problems is sought through team rather than individual effort because the team can bring a greater number of resources (skills, knowledge, information) to bear on the task, and thus presumably arrive at a better outcome than can one professional acting alone. The price for this improvement in outcome is a loss in efficiency due to the process of the group itself. This decrease in efficiency has been termed "process loss" (Steiner, 1972). For example, five professionals meeting for one hour cannot necessarily produce what one of them working alone could accomplish in five hours. This is because only part of the team's time and effort is spent in actual problem-solving activities; the rest of the time may be devoted to team interaction and team maintenance activities.

Most of the team activities will focus on providing clients with needed services. However, some time will be spent dealing with organizational matters and in activities aimed at one's professional colleagues. Thus the team member may find it necessary to attend meetings of the social work service or the psychology department. These meetings may be either task-related (for example, making decisions about work assignments or departmental policy) or maintenance-oriented (for example, clarifying roles or leadership within the department). Often the team member will be called on to participate in various activities, such as committee meetings and administrative assignments, that focus primarily on the organization rather than on specific clients. For example, initiating a team approach in a hospital or reorganizing from a departmental to a unit system will temporarily require considerable time and energy that might otherwise be spent in direct service to clients. Such organizational activities are likely to be task-related but can also involve some maintenance variables. For example, an overly rigid, authoritarian administration may lead to a reduction in task-related activities while the staff deals with its own internal morale problems.

In short, some of the team's resources may be used in activities related to professional and organizational goals, but the major team effort will be devoted to serving clients. The remainder of this chapter examines task-related, client-centered team activities.

OBSERVING THE TEAM CONFERENCE

One of the major problems in the study of teams is the lack of empirical data based on the systematic observation of team interaction. Most of the descriptive information presently available consists of reports by individual team participants in medical settings who describe in rather general terms what their team does and how it is organized. There have been few attempts by outside observers to examine team functioning. Yet this kind of systematic observation is necessary if some of the major parameters of team functioning are to be identified.

Although many team activities (such as collecting data about the patient and implementing treatment procedures) are carried out by individual team members, most teams engage in face-to-face interaction on a regular basis. These team meetings, case conferences, or staffings offer an excellent opportunity to observe team interaction and often highlight the roles, status, and power relationships within the team.

In order to explore the variables involved in these interactions, a series of observations were made of case conferences by teams operating in a variety of organizational settings. Drawing upon the concepts of Flanders (1967, 1970), Hare (1976), Bales (1950a, 1950b, 1955) and others concerned with category systems for observing human interaction, the authors designed a recording method specifically suited for the observation of team decision-making processes. The Team Observation Protocol (TOP) evolved from a series of observations of progress, consultation, and disposition staffings in medical and psychiatric settings, schools, and rehabilitation centers. Less complex than some of the other category systems, the TOP can be used to describe what goes on in the team session, compare teams in various institutional settings, or help a team's efforts toward self-evaluation.

The Team Observation Protocol (TOP)

The TOP is used to categorize the major statements of team members to identify who participates in the team discussion, what kind of statements are made by the various professionals, and how a decision is reached by the team. Seven categories of statements are used: Client, Team, Questions, Information, Interpretation, Alternatives, and Decisions. The TOP does not attempt to collect verbatim recordings of participants' statements or record nonverbal behavior. Nonverbal expressions (nodding, frowning, pointing, touching, etc.) may be noted anecdotally, but there is no attempt to categorize them.

In recording the verbal activities of the team, each participant is usually given a number and is identified by profession and sex. Responses of team members are numbered and recorded in one of the seven categories. Responses are numbered in the sequence in which they occur, so it is possible to reconstruct the sequence of the statements if this is desirable. If only frequency data are required, checks rather than numbers may be used; however, numbering in sequence gives far more information with little extra effort. Statements are recorded only once, regardless of length, unless the speaker moves to a new category of response. For example, the respondent may begin to report by sharing *information* about the client and conclude the statement by asking a *question* of another team member. This statement would be recorded once in each of the two categories. On the other hand,

---

Table 6-1 Recording Rules for the Team Observation Protocol

1. Each participant is identified by profession and sex and given a code number.
2. Only verbal statements are recorded.
3. Statements are recorded in numerical sequence (unless only frequency data are required).
4. Each statement is recorded by category and participant.
5. Each response is recorded only once regardless of length, unless there is a change in response category.
6. Each change in category is recorded as a new response.
7. Each change in respondent is recorded as a new response.

if the speaker's statement consisted of a long report of information about the client, this statement would be coded only once, even if it continued for five or ten minutes. Thus each statement is recorded every time there is a change of category or respondent. Since all the responses are numbered in sequence, the number of the last response reflects the total number of statements recorded during the session. The general recording rules are summarized in Table 6-1.

Categories of the TOP

Table 6-2 describes the seven statement categories. The TOP focuses greater attention on the cognitive, task-related aspects of team interaction than on affective, nonverbal elements. Only two categories are concerned with affective statements: Categories 1 and 2 which include affective statements about the client and

Table 6-2 Category Descriptions of the Team Observation Protocol

Category	Description
1. Client	All affective statements (+ or −) regarding the client. Neutral statements about the client are coded in categories 3-7; category 1 includes only statements revealing an emotional reaction to the client, such as hostile or joking references to the client.
2. Team	All affective statements (+ or −) about the team or a team member. Neutral statements about the team would be coded in categories 3-7; category 1 includes emotional reactions to the team itself or to another team member. It includes joking, laughing, or hostile remarks.
3. Questions	All statements asking for information, suggestions, or opinions, or requesting reports.
4. Information	All statements giving factual information, dealing only with what is observed, without interpretation.
5. Interpretation	All statements which give an opinion or interpretation, going beyond empirical data to make inferences about what has been observed.
6. Alternatives	All statements which suggest alternatives, explore or compare possible courses of action.
7. Decisions	All statements which deal directly with the final decision — expressing, clarifying, or elaborating the decision reached.

about other team members or the team as a whole. The other five categories focus on the tasks in which the team is involved: sharing information, drawing interpretations or hypotheses from that information, exploring the various alternatives available to the team, and finally, deciding on a course of action. Category 3, *Questions,* is a frequently used category in most team conferences, as team members seek information and opinions during the decision-making process.

Using the TOP

Figure 6-2 illustrates the recording method and the categories of the TOP as used in a fictional case conference. To simplify the example, only the profession of the participants and the response categories are included, and only a limited number of statements are reported.

This hypothetical case represents a team decision concerning a weekend home visit for a hospitalized psychiatric patient. Discussion is initiated by the physician who asks for a report by the nurse concerning the client's behavior on the ward (Response 1). Following the nurse's report (2), the physician asks the social worker for a report (3), and she replies with factual information regarding the client's history (4) and her opinion about the home situation (5). The physician asks a question (6), and the social worker responds with additional information (7). The psychologist's report is requested by the physician (8), and the psychologist describes the patient's test performance (9), interprets the patient's test scores (10), and suggests a course of action (11). The social worker asks a question (12). The physician replies, explaining the dynamics behind the patient's present symptoms (13) and discussing the possibility of a home visit (14). The social worker also comments regarding the pros and cons of the home visit (15), and the physician states, "Well, I think we should let him try a visit this weekend and see what happens" (16). The psychologist indicates that he feels positively about the client (17), and the physician concludes the discussion by reaffirming the decision (18).

Statements can be summarized by category and by participant (or by profession if several members of the same profession are present) and can be analyzed in a number of ways. For example, long staffings on a particular client can be broken into thirds or halves and the types of statements in each part compared. It may be found that the first third of the case conference will focus on questions and information statements, the middle third on interpretations, and the last third on alternatives and decisions. The numbering of responses facilitates the analysis of the interaction sequence. Although the example given in Figure 6-2 is too brief for this kind of analysis, even a cursory examination of the data suggests that in this particular case the physician is playing an active leadership role in the decision process, while the nurse is quite passive. The physician begins and ends the discussion and asks most of the questions.

Figure 6-2 Example of TOP Record

PARTICIPANTS	1. Client	2. Team	3. Questions	4. Information	5. Interpretation	6. Alternatives	7. Decisions	TOTAL
Physician			1-3 6-8		13	14	16-18	8
Nurse				2				1
Social Worker			12	4-7	5	15		5
Psychologist	17+			9	10	11		4
TOTAL	1+	0	5	4	3	3	2	18

At this point it may be helpful to look at some case conferences and see how teams actually operate in such sessions. The following examples are composite descriptions of observations made by the authors in a number of different settings. Although these examples are fictional, they are representative of observations of actual teams.

TEAM CONFERENCE A

The first example is a medical staffing at a large hospital. We have arranged the visit in advance and have asked permission to take notes during the staffing.

10:00 a.m.   It is a bright October day as we arrive at the facility where we are to observe a team conference. As we approach the reception desk the atmosphere is one of crisp efficiency. We are directed to the conference room where the staffing is to be held. It is a large comfortable room with a T-shaped conference table in the center. Three other tables are arranged on the periphery of the room. A coffee urn and pastries are arranged on a table against one wall.

10:15   Two nurses enter the room, they glance briefly at us and begin arranging a number of large looseleaf case books at the head of the table. A third nurse enters, moves to inspect the arrangement of the case books, notices us, and frowns slightly. She moves quickly to where we are seated; we rise. She introduces herself, as do we. Our legitimacy is established; we are offered coffee. We are no longer noticed.

10:20   The third nurse lifts the phone from its wall hook and speaks briefly. Almost as an echo the page is heard, "Dr. Johnson's case conference will start in 10 minutes." A middle-aged woman enters with her arms full of folders. She takes her place at the head table and arranges her folders and her pens. We learn later that she is an administrative aide.

10:25   The page is heard again: "Dr. Johnson's case conference will begin in five minutes." People start to arrive. For the most part they are young, and a majority are female. A few get coffee; most do not. They begin taking seats. Some begin to review notes; some begin to write. We are briefly noted by a physical therapist who pulls an extra chair to the table where we are sitting. We are again ignored.

10:31   Dr. Johnson enters and glances at us briefly as he takes his place at the center of the head table, Nurse Three and One to his left. A sentence from Dr. Johnson to Nurse Three, a few words in return; we are legitimate again.

10:32   Nurse Three hands Dr. Johnson a case book. Dr. Johnson begins. The case is a male, amputee, 73 years old. Other information from the case record. Then, Johnson: "Nursing?" Nursing gives information. There is a brief exchange with Johnson showing agreement with nursing's information about the case. Nursing expands on the information. Johnson responds with agreement.

"Social Work?" She gives information with no response from Johnson.

"PT?" PT gives information; Johnson responds with a question; there is another exchange of comments. PT gives five separate statements of information; Johnson asks three questions and gives information three times. PT has also given three statements of interpretation. Johnson ends the exchange with further information and an interpretation and a short joke. Then back to business.

"OT?" Gives information.

"ADL?" Gives information.

"Psychology?" Gives information.

Johnson asks a rhetorical question and answers with his opinion. The case is finished. Like card players throwing in their hands, each of the participants throws a small slip of paper to the center of the table. The slips contain each team member's goals for the patient.

10:41   Johnson says, "Review in two weeks."

Total elapsed time — nine minutes, during which time 34 separate statements were made: 19 by Johnson, 3 by Nursing, 8 by PT, and one each by all other professions. With the exception of PT and Johnson, the other participants confined their responses to giving information. When the PT did give an opinion, Johnson followed up by asking for further interpretation.

10:42   The next case begins. Johnson introduces. "Nursing?" "Social Work?" "PT?" "OT?" "ADL?" "Psychology?" — on through the morning. As individuals complete their cases, they leave and are replaced by someone from a side table. The seating arrangement does not vary; the order of reporting remains the same. People enter and leave the room with the exception of the physician and the administrative aide. All is calm, efficient, and without visible emotion. Suddenly, an empty chair. The PT has left the center table and has not been replaced. Everyone looks at our table where two PTs are sitting. They look uncomfortable, but neither moves. Johnson asks which PT is assigned to the next case. One PT responds "Williams." "Page Mr. Williams." But Nurse Three is already at the phone: "Mr. Williams is wanted in Dr. Johnson's case conference immediately." There is even a slight hint of stridence in the usually smooth voice of the page operator. One of the PTs at our table leaves the room. "Nursing?" "Social Work?" "OT?"

11:50   All look uncomfortably at the empty chair that Johnson has skipped in the litany. "ADL?" "Psychology?" Johnson makes his decision. The goals are thrown to the center of the table. Williams arrives and sits down. "PT?" Williams reports on the case that has already been concluded. Johnson makes no response. There is an air of discomfort in the room, a result of the unspoken reprimand.

12:00   The next case begins. The time passes. Some individuals have been in the room for the whole two hours. Some have been in and out and back again. Another M.D. wanders in, gets some coffee, and sits at one of the side tables for a while. Then she leaves. The tempo has not changed all morning, with the exception of the Williams incident. Then a case is announced: Mr. Jones, male, 52, hip surgery. As the name is announced there is a noticeable increase in interest. A groan comes from at least one of the participants. Johnson pretends not to notice this, but by his posture and demeanor you can see that he has. The reports start. "Nursing?" Nursing gives a long report of Jones' transgressions, his intransigence about taking medication, his surliness to the nurses, his insistence on doing things his way, his dissatisfaction with the food, his friend's successful attempt to smuggle in a bottle of gin and the subsequent disruption. "Social Work?" Social Work begins to report, but discipline has broken down. Each of the services rushes to contribute a tale concerning the trouble Jones has caused. At times two or more services compete for the floor, each trying to outdo the other with a report on Jones. Finally the uproar subsides. There is an embarrassed pause and one senses a slight amount of discomfort in the group; they have overstepped the boundary. Psychology speaks; "He did do well on his test last week." This breaks the silence. Each service contributes something positive about Jones. They atone for transgressing professional bounds. The discussion becomes more professional. Discipline is restored and a decision is reached — reevaluate in two weeks. Slips are passed to the center of the table. The next case begins.

1:14 p.m.   The last case is over. Someone gathers the slips of paper from the center of the table, to be sorted and recorded in the case book. Nurses One and Two collect the case books. Johnson is speaking to the administrative aide. Other staffers have left quickly. We thank Dr. Johnson. He says, "Anytime," and we leave.

TEAM CONFERENCE B

Now let us visit a rather different facility. This agency is a residential treatment center for clients with mental health problems. Late afternoon, around 4 p.m., we arrive at the front door of a large house on a quiet residential street. The street is no longer "fashionable," and many of the older houses have been converted to apartments for young married couples or singles. A few new condominiums have replaced some of the older houses. We see a sign directing us to enter through the double doors which still have their cut glass windows of former, grander times.

The hall and living room have the feel of a fraternity house; however, in this case it is co-ed. Several young people are lounging in the living room, a few are seen moving up the stairs with mop and pail. We stop at a small reception desk, and the young man asks what we want in a direct, no-nonsense manner. We are to meet with the director. We are checked out on the intercom and motioned up the stairs.

The director's office is a converted bedroom on the second floor. He is on the phone, his feet on the desk. A few olive drab filing cabinets and a pair of wooden chairs complete the decor. We are waved to the chairs. After the phone call he questions us briefly as to our purpose; then he offers a description of the facility.

4:15	The team meeting that was to have started at 4 p.m. is about to begin. We move across the hall to another converted bedroom. It is furnished with several overstuffed chairs of uncertain vintage, an end table, a phone, a sofa that is losing its springs, and a number of brown folding metal chairs. There is a worn imitation Oriental rug on the floor.
4:18	People begin to drift into the room. We are for the most part ignored. The director leaves to take another phone call.
4:20	There are now nine persons seated around the periphery of the room. They range in age from 25 to 35 and are equally divided between men and women. The director returns and opens the meeting. We are introduced and the purpose of our visit is explained. The staff persons are introduced by name and role; there are three counselors, a vocational specialist, a nurse, a supervisor of counseling, a supervisor of residential services, a counseling student, the director, and his assistant.
4:25	The first case begins when the director says, "What about Jerry?" What follows is a progress review of a particular patient; there is no particular order to the responses. Discussion ensues for about ten minutes. The director does not intervene in the discussion until 22 statements have been made by others. In the next 10 minutes he asks seven questions and gives two statements of interpretation. The most active speaker in the group is the supervisor of residential services. Others join in the discussion freely, but the director and the supervisor of residential services make the most comments. There are some digressions; Jerry, it seems, has been up and down several "levels" in the agency, and some members feel that as he gets more responsibility he also becomes more manipulative. Now he is assigned to cook for the residence. There are groans from several of the counselors (who must eat with the residents). The decision is made, however, and Jerry is promoted to chief cook. Two more clients are discussed, each with a particular set of problems: probation, the police, getting along with others in the facility, problems with the staff. The interrelatedness of residents' problems is reflected in the discussion, which switches focus from one client to another with great rapidity. The director takes a phone call in the conference room, but the discussion goes on. In fact, a decision is made while he is still on the phone.
5:00	The director asks, "Is there anything else?" There are a few individual questions, but people are already leaving the room. The meeting is over.

These two examples present some striking contrasts as well as some similarities. First, the marked differences in the physical environments seem to emphasize the more basic differences in the overall atmosphere of the two settings. In the first example, the physician is clearly the team leader and the most active participant in making the final decision. In the second example, team leadership is more diffuse; indeed, several members seem to assume a leadership role from time to time during the session.

The medical team appears to be formal, well organized, efficient, and somewhat impersonal in its operation; while the second team appears to be more casual, informal, and more personal in its interaction. Yet in both team meetings we see essentially the same activities: reporting information, making hypotheses about the client, and reaching some decision. Both hypothetical teams have clear communication networks and well established operating procedures, and both attempt to provide coordinated services for their clients. Thus both groups appear to meet the criteria for teams as proposed in Chapter One.

The Team Observation Protocol has been used by the authors in observing a number of different kinds of teams. The two examples cited above were based on elements from several of those observations. It may be helpful to examine the TOP results from some of those teams.

RESULTS OF TEAM OBSERVATIONS

Team conferences were observed in several settings, including medical rehabilitation units, alcohol/drug rehabilitation centers, residential schools for the developmentally disabled, and day schools. The team meetings were staffings of one or more clients, involving decisions about such matters as treatment, discharge, or home visits. Results of nine team observations are summarized in Table 6-3. Since interest was focused on the decision process itself, recording was confined to the case presentations. Informal interactions before and after the team conference and between case presentations were not recorded in these observations. This probably accounts for the low percentage of responses about the team or team members (Category 2). Each case was recorded separately, from the introduction of the client to the concluding comment. The time spent on a single case varied from two or three minutes (this usually occurred with cases presented at the end of a meeting, when only a quick progress report was given), to two or three hours (when the entire meeting was devoted to discussion of one client). The number of cases presented in a single session ranged from 1 to 15, and the length of the sessions varied from 42 to 159 minutes. The number of team members participating in the discussion of any one case ranged from 3 to 20 (however, not every team member contributed to every case), and the number of members present at each of the nine team meetings ranged from 7 to 25.

Table 6-3 Team Observation Protocol Summaries of Nine Teams

TEAM		1. CLIENT	2. TEAM	3. QUEST.	4. INFORM.	5. INTERP.	6. ALTERN.	7. DECIS.	TOTAL
				STATEMENT CATEGORIES					
1. Medical Rehabilitation 10 cases	N=	9	11	94	100	58	30	33	335
	%=	2.7	3.3	28.1	29.9	17.3	9.0	9.8	
2. Drug/Alcohol 4 cases	N=	30	10	42	74	47	24	10	237
	%=	12.7	4.2	17.7	31.2	19.8	10.1	4.2	
3. Medical Rehabilitation 12 cases	N=	17	0	108	126	85	45	22	403
	%=	4.2	0	26.8	31.3	21.1	11.2	5.5	
4. Medical Rehabilitation 15 cases	N=	3	2	74	89	60	27	9	264
	%=	1.1	0.7	28.0	33.7	22.7	10.2	3.4	
5. Residential School 1 case	N=	14	0	97	91	63	17	12	294
	%=	4.8	0	33.0	31.0	21.4	5.8	4.1	
6. Medical Rehabilitation 10 cases	N=	5	3	73	81	39	14	18	233
	%=	2.1	1.3	31.3	34.8	16.7	6.0	7.7	
7. Residential School 1 case	N=	6	0	30	40	45	4	3	128
	%=	4.7	0	23.4	31.3	35.2	3.1	2.3	
8. Residential School 1 case	N=	1	2	44	95	32	15	6	195
	%=	0.5	1.0	22.6	48.7	16.4	7.7	3.1	
9. School (Day) 1 case	N=	2	1	35	40	53	17	3	151
	%=	1.3	.7	23.2	26.5	35.1	11.3	2.0	
Total	N=	87	29	597	736	482	193	116	2240
	%=	3.9	1.3	26.7	32.9	21.5	8.6	5.2	

Responses by Category

Table 6-3 confirms what was illustrated in the hypothetical examples given above: the team conference tends to be quite task-oriented, with relatively little byplay among participants during the case presentations. The total percentages of *Client* and *Team* statements across the nine teams are only 3.9 percent and 1.3 percent respectively; thus, almost 95 percent of the statements made in these observations were task-related and concerned directly with the client. The largest percentage of total responses (32.9) are in the *Information* category. In six of the nine teams this was the most frequently used category, while *Interpretation* was most frequent in two teams, and *Questions* in one team. Together these three categories (Questions, Information, and Interpretation) account for 81.1 percent of all statements recorded in the nine teams observed.

As noted earlier, the high proportion of task-related statements reflects an artifact of the procedure used — that is, recording only during actual case discussions and not before, after, or between case presentations. It is also possible that the presence of the observers motivated the participants to "stick to the task" and reduced the amount of tangential discussion. Nevertheless, the high percentage of statements devoted to sharing information and hypotheses about the client is striking, and suggests that at least the particular teams observed by the authors were quite task oriented, with relatively little emphasis on group maintenance activities. It is speculated that similar results would be obtained with other teams in other kinds of team settings; that, in fact, one of the major characteristics of human service and health-related teams is their focus on task-related activities.

While these results with the TOP give us some preliminary information about the decision processes used by teams, much more empirical data about team interaction must be collected if we are to fully understand the dynamics of a team conference. It should also be noted that much team interaction occurs outside the team meeting itself, in informal consultations between team members. We will examine more fully some of the factors affecting team dynamics in the next chapter.

TEAM TASKS AND RELATED ACTIVITIES

What emerges from the two descriptions of team conferences is a consistent sequence of activities as the team carries out its various tasks relative to the client. While the individual team member may perform certain tasks such as measuring blood pressure or writing progress notes, the team itself engages in other activities — e.g., integrating the information presented, making decisions about the course of treatment, and evaluating its outcome.

Figure 6-3 shows how the task-related activities of a team can be divided between those carried out by the individual team members and those performed by the team as a whole. Five major tasks related to client service are identified: (1) data collection, (2) assessment, (3) decision making, (4) treatment, and (5) evaluation. Some of the typical team and individual activities are indicated for each type of task. For example, during assessment, individual team members will report and interpret the data they have collected. Assessment activities for the team involve integrating the information provided in the reports of various team members, suggesting a diagnosis, and refining the tentative goals that had been set for the client. Thus the team, through team conferences and other activities, coordinates the work of the professionals involved in the case. Now let us examine how the team carries out the five tasks identified in Figure 6-3.

Data Collection

One of the major tasks of the team is the collecting and sharing of information about the client. Generally, each team member is responsible for gathering certain specific information and perhaps measuring some aspect of the client. As a result of this division of labor in the collection of information about the client, we often speak in terms of "educational data," "social history data," "medical results," and "personality measurement," as though the client could be divided into parts and each part measured separately. We sometimes lose sight of the "whole person" and forget that categories such as physical, mental, social, and educational have been created for our own convenience. Such categories are not inherent in the client, who functions as a whole being. It is part of the function of the team to reintegrate and reinterpret the *whole* of the evidence or data gathered by a number of team professionals.

It should also be kept in mind that the data collected includes only that which can be *observed* from the physical properties of the client or his or her behavior or interaction with the milieu. Anything that is not directly observable is *inferred* from observable indicators. Such inferences usually involve hypotheses about the current status of the client or predictions about the client's future status. For example, a physician measures an individual's height and weight, finds that her weight exceeds the norm for her height, and advises the person to lose weight. In this case, the doctor has inferred that the client will be "healthier" if her weight is closer to the norm for her height and age. This inference is based on the frequency of health problems associated with overweight in other persons. However, it should be pointed out that this is only a statement of probability and is not necessarily true for this particular client. Similarly, the doctor who finds an abnormally high white blood cell count could infer that there may be an infection, but might be unable to predict where the infection is located. However, when this sign is coupled with pain and tenderness in the lower right abdomen, the doctor may well predict an infected appendix. In this case, the doctor is again using a predictive model based on probability statements.

Figure 6-3 Individual and Team Activities

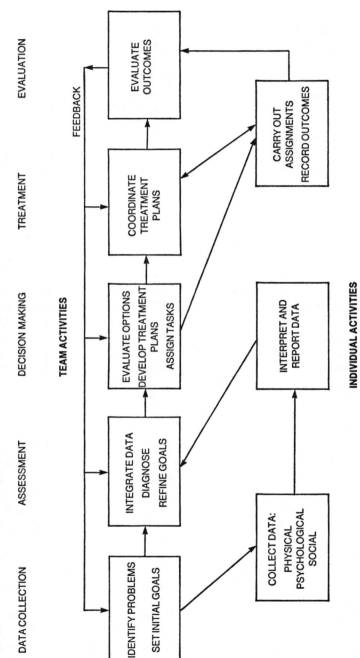

Use of Norms

In many cases, information collected about the client or measurements taken by team members are compared with the average or typical measures of a larger population. Such average scores or measures are called *norms.* Often a measure taken of an individual client has little meaning unless such a comparison is made. Only then can it be determined that the client is average, higher, or lower on the particular measure than persons in the norm group.

However, the use of norms for making comparisons can present several difficulties. One problem is the lack of clear definition and identification of the comparison group. Another related problem is finding an adequate sample of the population. Of course, it is clearly inappropriate to compare the achievement test results of a fourth grade boy against the scores made by a group of eighth graders, and then conclude that the boy is "below average" because his scores are much lower than the norm group. Yet there are instances in which equally inappropriate comparisons have been made. Since some measures may be related to certain factors such as sex, age, geographical location, education, socioeconomic status, and ethnic or cultural background, many questions have been raised concerning the population from which particular norms have been derived and whether these norms are sufficiently representative to support the kinds of decisions usually based on them. Failure to use appropriate norms may discriminate unfairly against particular individuals or groups (such as those of different social classes or persons with physical and medical handicaps). Although this problem is most significant with psychological and educational measures, it can also apply to physical measures. For example, charts representing average or "normal" height and weight measures based on data gathered in the United States would be inappropriate to use with Japanese populations. In short, norms must be used with full recognition of the particular characteristics of the population on which the norms were based.

Agencies and institutions often develop their own set of norms or baselevel data that reflects the particular population at hand. Even when this is not done formally and systematically, norms are adapted informally by agency personnel and reflected in statements such as, "We almost never see a case like this" or "Most of our patients do not do well with that type of test." Teams that have worked together will quickly identify those clients who are "different" from the usual client served by the team.

Sources of Error in Data Collection

All data collection involves error. The team members who report information based on measurements of the client cannot be absolutely accurate, and even if they were we would never know it. Some measurement error is always assumed to exist. This can be easily demonstrated with even a relatively simple measure such as body temperature. Ask several persons to take and record the body temperature of the same patient, and the results are likely to show variation due to error in measurement. Complex measures (psychological, educational) are even more subject to error than are physical measures.

Several sources of measurement error have been described including: observer error, error in the instrument, and error arising from variation in what is being measured (Walker and Lev, 1953; Noll, 1965). Observer error refers to individual differences between observers; that is, two observers will often "see" things quite differently. Observer error also includes variation within the same observer. "A single observer's own readings will commonly be found to vary from one observation to the next, even though the actual conditions are unchanged" (Noll, 1965, p. 9). The psychologist suffering from a cold or headache may come up with different data than that found when feeling well.

Instrument error results from the fact that no device, no matter how well calibrated, is perfectly accurate. There is sometimes variation between instruments and occasionally within the same instrument.

Finally, there is the error attributable to variation in the individual being measured (or in his environment). For example, measurement error is likely to result when taking a patient's oral temperature immediately after he has swallowed hot soup, or giving an intelligence test in a cold and uncomfortable room. In these cases measurement error stems from the variability of the patient's response. Often the team member is unaware of conditions that immediately preceded the testing or measuring period — conditions that might have a significant effect on the consistency of the client's responses. Often team members who take similar measurements at different times find quite different results with the same client. This can lead to puzzling contradictions in the information reported at the case conference, and the team must either collect additional data or arrive at some explanation that resolves the inconsistencies.

Assessment

Following the collection of data and the measurement of pertinent variables, the data must be organized, summarized, and interpreted if it is to be useful to the team in assessing the status of the client. Assessment can be regarded as "the systematic collection, organization, and interpretation of information about a person and his situation" (Sundberg and Tyler, 1962, p. 81).

One characteristic of the team approach is a comprehensive view of all aspects of the client's functioning, rather than a narrow focus on a single aspect. In rehabilitation, for example, the team approach has long been popular, in part because the psychological and social aspects of the patient so clearly affect the process of physical rehabilitation. Since one person cannot adequately measure and interpret all aspects of the patient's functioning, the team works together to make a valid assessment of the client.

Child guidance and mental health clinics are two other settings where the team approach has been widely used. Here the clients are likely to have interrelated problems that cannot be easily separated into physical, psychological, educational, and social components. Bedwetting in a 12-year-old boy, for example, is often the result of combined physical, psychological, and social (or family) factors, and each component must be assessed and integrated before treatment can be implemented.

Usually team members collect and interpret the information their profession regards as within its province. The information is shared with the team through a written report, a verbal presentation, or both. Sometimes, of course, there is overlap, and two professionals may ask some of the same questions and collect similar data. This is a potential source of conflict if one professional feels that the information somehow "belongs" to her or his profession and that another professional is encroaching on that territory.

Once the data has been collected, the measures taken, and the questions asked, the information must be organized and summarized into a more usable form. For example, data collected through the Minnesota Multiphasic Personality Inventory (MMPI) consists of answers to over 500 questions. Such a mass of data is almost unusable, and therefore MMPI results are usually summarized as scores on less than a dozen scales. In the same way, statisticians have shown us how thousands of numbers can be summarized by just two numbers: the mean and the standard deviation (measures of the average score and of the amount of "spread" of the scores).

Once the data has been summarized in a useful form, the professional attempts to "make sense" out of it. Sometimes interpretation actually begins with the process of data collection. Despite attempts to reduce the subjectivity in our observations and data gathering instruments, certain biases inherent in the human observer cannot be completely eliminated. Weitz (1964) has pointed out how selection and abstraction distort the information conveyed and the interpretations made in the interaction of a counselor and client. His point is relevant to the collection and interpretation of information by other professionals as well. The steps identified by Weitz are:

1. The client participates in some event.
2. Out of all the elements in the event, the client selects some; these he perceives and responds to.
3. Out of all the responses made by the client in the situation, he selects some; these he reports to the counselor.
4. The counselor listens to the client, and while he is listening, he symbolically projects some of his own similar experiences into the client's description.

5. Out of this total description — including the counselor's projections — the counselor selects some elements; these he perceives and responds to by drawing inferences and formulating structures.

6. Out of all of these inferences and structures, the counselor selects some; these he reports. This report by the counselor, involving high-order abstractions in some cases far removed from the original event, is his tentative problem identification or diagnosis. (Weitz, 1964, p. 81).

Thus the final report of the professional may contain a great many higher-order abstractions, "in some cases far removed from the original event" as Weitz indicates. In this way the professional's perception of the client may be biased by his or her own past experience and training. The professional could be influenced by previous experiences with other clients ("Oh yes, that sounds very much like the symptoms Mrs. Smith reported") as well as by the particular approach or theoretical viewpoint to which the professional subscribes. Differences in viewpoint *between* professions may be so great that they use very different "jargon" to describe the same event. However, even *within* a profession there may be very different perceptions based on divergent theoretical viewpoints, and this can lead the team member to focus on different events or interpret them differently.

Ideally, then, assessment consists of collecting objective information with a minimum of inference, and then interpreting that data and forming hypotheses regarding the client. As we have seen, however, the process is usually not so simple, and there will always be some degree of error in data collection and assessment procedures. It is important that the professional not make premature inferences and conclusions during the period of information gathering. When the team member feels sufficient data has been collected, it is summarized, organized in a coherent way, and finally, interpreted.

It should be noted that data collection does not then cease — it continues so long as the client is in treatment. The information gathering and assessment process is an iterative one, with new information giving new meaning to what has been previously learned. For example, a patient presents certain signs and symptoms, several hypotheses are suggested, and a tentative diagnosis is made. Various additional tests are then made, and this new information either confirms or contradicts the hypotheses and the diagnosis. In the latter case, new hypotheses will suggest themselves and more tests may be run to confirm the new diagnosis. The process of assessment is therefore a continuing team activity.

Decision Making

Another major function of the team as indicated in Figure 6-3 is decision making. In some cases decisions represent a consensus of the total membership of the team; in other cases, decision making is regarded as primarily the responsibility of one member of the team. Nevertheless, it is a *team* task, even if the team leader or some other member regularly makes the final decision.

Elements of Decision Making

There are two key concepts involved in the decision process: choice and alternatives. The option to choose among two or more alternatives is crucial to decision making. If either element is absent — that is, if the individual is not in a position to choose or if only one course of action is available — then there is no decision to be made. Teams often complain that although a considerable portion of the team meeting is devoted to an exploration of various alternatives, the team really does not have the authority to choose between them. The decision has already been made.

In any decision situation there must be an identification of the nature and range of options available. In many decision situations the decision maker must limit the range of alternatives to examine in coming to a decision. This in itself constitutes a prior choice, since some very attractive or viable alternatives may be eliminated. The importance of this initial narrowing of choices is often not recognized, even though it may in fact represent the *most* important decision. Sometimes one may not be aware that such narrowing has occurred. For example, the acceptance of one theoretical framework is an effective way of limiting alternatives, but this may occur quite naturally, without extensive deliberation.

This idea is illustrated by the concept of the decision tree. A decision tree attempts to map the consequences of a decision. As can be seen in the example in Figure 6-4, as one moves through the tree and reaches certain decisions, other possibilities are deleted, thereby truncating the tree. Theoretically, a decision tree might be constructed that would illustrate *all* of the possible decision consequences from an initial decision point. It has been pointed out, however, that the decision tree for evaluating a single opening chess move would consist of 10^{120} branches (Steen, 1975). It is clear that the professional's role is to prune the tree to the point where it is manageable by eliminating as many of the unfruitful branches as possible.

Another element that should be noted from the decision tree is that the impact of decisions and subsequent actions is sequential. Prior decisions alter the status of the person and thus alter the information upon which subsequent decisions are based. It is important to recognize this when dealing with a client over a long period of time or when evaluating previous decisions made by other professionals. Decision trees illustrate that decisions may lead down irreversible paths, thus making a seemingly unimportant decision crucial to the eventual outcome.

For example, a casual decision to cancel a dental appointment because "something came up," may later lead to a choice between the loss of a tooth or root canal work. With a medical patient, the choice to use a particular medication may later rule out the use of other drugs.

Figure 6-4 Example of a Decision Tree

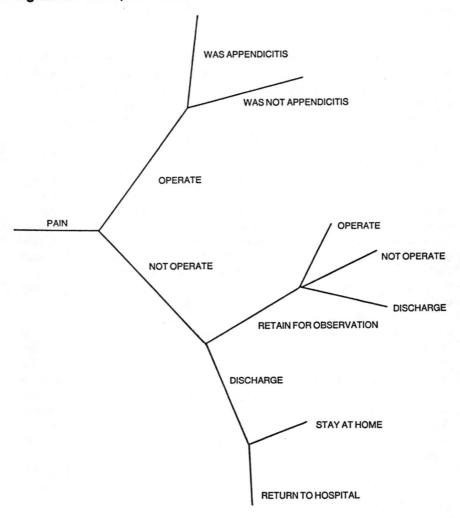

Ideally, a decision maker functions rationally; that is, he or she decides on the basis of an evaluation of the data and uses that data to reduce the chance of error. Unfortunately, humans do not always act rationally. Furthermore, the individual who is able to make relatively rational choices in one situation may become quite irrational in another area.

Despite the interest in decision processes, we still know very little about how people actually make decisions. This is partly because much of the empirical data about decisions comes from laboratory situations where the risks are quite different from those inherent in *real* decision making. One fact is quite clear however: individuals react very differently to a decision task. We are all familiar with the decision maker who must have "more data" before a decision can be made, even when the available data seem abundant to the point of redundancy. There is also the individual who puts off a decision until events take over and a decision is no longer possible. These reactions often occur because of an aversion to risk. Since most real decisions of any importance present an element of risk *for the decision maker*, delaying and avoiding a decision may be seen as an attempt to escape from risk. Collecting additional data may help reduce risk up to a point, but when it becomes a ritualistic response to any decision, it is no more than a rather thinly disguised avoidance mechanism.

This behavior is often reflected in the case conference. For example, a social worker may indicate, "We don't have enough information right now to take any action. We should wait until I have spoken to the family." Or the nurse may indicate, "We should wait until next week when Dr. Smith comes in. Let's see what information he has before acting." This reluctance to make decisions may be seen by other team members as resistance or opposition to the team's decisions. Of course, if several team members take such a position, decision making may virtually cease.

Decision Error

Earlier in this chapter we discussed the concept of error in measurement. Let us now examine how error occurs in decision making and how to keep error at a minimum. Scheff (1963) has offered an interesting analysis of the role of error in medical diagnosis using the statistical concept of hypothesis testing. Two types of errors in statistical decision making have been identified, *Type 1 errors* and *Type 2 errors*. Simply stated, Type 1 errors are those in which a true hypothesis is rejected, while Type 2 errors are those in which a hypothesis that is really false is accepted as true.

This concept is well known to everyone familiar with the instruction to the jury that to be convicted of a crime an individual must be found guilty "beyond a reasonable doubt." That is, it is more important to avoid convicting an innocent person (rejecting a true hypothesis of innocence) than to set free a guilty one (accepting a false hypothesis of innocence).

Scheff sees an analogous situation in medical decision making. It is often assumed that disease is progressive and to avoid or delay treatment will be harmful to the patient. Thus a Type 1 error (rejecting a hypothesis of illness when the patient is indeed sick) is to be avoided whenever possible. The consequences of Type 2 errors (accepting the hypothesis of illness when the patient is actually well) are seen as far less serious. The patient may be inconvenienced, may have unnecessary financial expenses, and in some cases may even suffer unnecessary pain and discomfort from diagnostic or operative procedures, but nevertheless, conservative decision making is generally regarded as "good medicine." It is only when the frequency of Type 2 errors becomes unduly large (as when numerous complaints are filed about unnecessary surgery) that the values underlying such medical decisions are called into question. The alternative outcomes in medical decision making are identified by Scheff:

> A physician who dismisses a patient who subsequently dies of a disease that should have been detected [Type 1 error] is not only subject to legal action for negligence and possible loss of license for incompetence, but also to moral condemnation. . . . Nothing remotely resembling this amount of moral and legal suasion is brought to bear for committing a Type 2 error. Indeed this error is sometimes seen as sound clinical practice, indicating a healthy conservative approach to medicine (Scheff, 1963, p. 99).

There are, of course, situations in which the medical expert will be particularly careful to guard against a Type 2 error. Where the medical treatment itself is extremely dangerous (as with some types of surgery), it is as important to avoid unnecessary treatment as to provide needed treatment. Treatment for rabies provides a good example of the dilemma of medical decision making. Suppose it is not certain whether the patient has actually been infected. Failure to treat when the patient has been infected (Type 1 error) means almost certain death. Yet rabies treatment itself carries a certain degree of risk as well as pain, so a Type 2 error may also be harmful to the patient.

There are several points to note. First, data used in medical decision making is not always clearcut and in many instances decisions are made on the basis of mere probabilities. Second, it is important to weigh the relative impact of various errors in each situation, since the risks vary from one situation to the next. Third, we have focused on the impact of error on the *client*, but it should be noted that error poses risks to the *decision makers* as well. For example, in misdiagnosing an illness the decision maker has made an error that could ruin his or her professional reputation and result in a suit for malpractice. On the other hand, an error that finds a person ill and a candidate for additional tests or consultations is not as risky since the decision is equivocal. The costs will probably not be catastrophic for any one patient and will not entail high risk to the decision maker. Thus, in high risk medical situations physicians tend to seek a conservative alternative in order to minimize the risks to themselves and to the patient. While this may sound like optimum practice, there is some question as to its social utility (in terms of the increased cost of treatment) and cost to individuals (in terms of increased pain and reduction of the quality of life for unnecessary periods of time).

The decision making process is an important aspect of the team approach. One advantage is that there is less likelihood that a decision made by one team member will obviate the decisions of other team members. In traditional arrangements staffpersons sometimes complain that patients are discharged before they have completed treatment or before follow-up arrangements have been made. Team decision making can help to prevent such problems.

In this section we have focused on decision making by individuals. The results of decision making in groups will be examined more closely in the next chapter.

Treatment

For many professionals the most important activity is the actual treatment itself. In this phase the team functions as a vehicle for coordinating the activities of the various professionals as they apply their particular expertise in the treatment of a client. The team *does not* usurp the functions of the individual professions, but rather serves to coordinate and mediate in implementing the plan of action.

In some instances this coordination involves the simultaneous treatment of the client. Resuscitation teams, surgical teams, and dental teams, for example, may treat the patient *as a team,* with all members actually working on the patient at the same time in a carefully coordinated series of moves. The more usual treatment, however, involves team members working individually but coordinating their actions through written plans, team meetings, or informal communication. The extent to which the treatment is provided as an integrated package depends then on the immediate problem that is being addressed.

Regardless of how treatment is provided, this phase of the team's efforts is often the most crucial, for it provides the means for changing the client's situation. However, if the earlier steps of data collection, assessment, and decision making have not been carried out in a careful and thorough manner, so as to provide the necessary groundwork, treatment activities may not be as effective as anticipated.

Evaluation

Evaluation of the outcomes of the team's efforts is an ongoing process that is a part of each of the activities described above. Has enough data been collected? What other information is needed? How can we account for this finding? Which alternative would lead to a better outcome for the patient? Is the new medication having the hoped-for effect? Team members are constantly receiving feedback and evaluating the effect of their actions on the client. A more formal evaluation of the effectiveness of decision making and treatment may come at the time of discharge or during follow-up. Evaluation will be discussed more fully in Chapter Eight.

Chapter 7

Team Dynamics

In Chapter Six we looked at *what* the team does — the activities by which the team carries out its tasks and attains its task-related goals. In this chapter we are interested in *how* the team conducts itself and in those activities that contribute to team maintenance. Since there has been little research dealing specifically with the dynamics of interdisciplinary teams, we will examine what has been learned about small group dynamics and see how those findings relate to the team.

Interest and research in the dynamics of small groups has accelerated rapidly in the last half century (Hare, 1976; Shaw, 1976). Social psychologists and others have conducted extensive research on the variables affecting group interaction and productivity, investigating such diverse topics as therapy and growth groups, T groups, juvenile groups, work groups, problem-solving groups, and decision-making groups. Some of this research has involved observations of existing groups in their natural settings; more often it has involved the creation of short-term experimental groups in laboratory situations. Although many questions regarding the operation of small groups remain unresolved, research with a variety of subjects and types of groups has led to the identification of a number of common factors. Five major characteristics that distinguish a "group" from a "collection of individuals" have been identified. "The members of the group are in *interaction* with one another. They share a common *goal* and set of *norms*, which give direction and limits to their activity. They also develop a set of *roles* and a *network of interpersonal attraction*, which serve to differentiate them from other groups" (Hare, 1976, p. 5). In looking at the team and how it functions, we will examine these characteristics and certain related concepts of group dynamics such as power, status, conformity, coalition formation, and size and composition of the team.

THE TEAM AS A SMALL GROUP

The teams with which this book is concerned are typically small groups of professionals who meet in face-to-face interaction with a common purpose. Such teams vary along a number of dimensions including size and composition, characteristics of members, physical setting, tasks to be performed, and type of interaction. Along with these characteristics that are shared with groups in general, interdisciplinary teams have certain unique attributes that should be noted. For example, as we have seen, teams are usually part of a larger institutional setting such as a school, a hospital, a clinic, or similar organization. Also, it is more likely that roles will be assigned on the basis of professional expertise or job title than by group consensus.

Teams do not usually emerge spontaneously as other small groups often do. Rather, membership in the team is usually a specific job responsibility, or may be so perceived. Thus team membership may be imposed from without, and this involuntary aspect of participation is likely to affect the individual's interaction within the team. Furthermore, the rewards for participation may also come from outside the team rather than from within it. Raises and promotions may be seen as rewards for being a "good" team member or a frequent participant.

On the other hand, outside factors may interfere with team performance if staffings or team meetings are seen as unrewarded and a "waste of time" so far as professional aspirations are concerned. The effect of outside pressures on the performance of individual team members and on performance of the team is a factor that deserves more study, and while it may be insignificant in controlled laboratory studies it appears to be crucial in the real-life team functioning.

Generally the team operates within certain other constraints imposed by the work setting and by the task itself. Frequency of meetings, stability of membership, and size of the team may be influenced by organizational or administrative factors. Unlike groups in which the leadership is selected by the group members, teams will often have formal leaders assigned by virtue of their position or professional status, although other informal leaders may emerge from the team itself. Related to this is the issue of autonomy — that is, the extent to which team decisions are put into action rather than being vetoed at another level. Such outcomes have impact not only on the decision-making process, but also on the continued involvement and motivation of team members.

Team members may also differ in the extent of their legal responsibility for the patient. As we pointed out in Chapter Six, decisions about real patients are necessarily different from decisions made in a laboratory experiment. The relationship of real life-threatening situations to group decision processes has not been clearly investigated.

TEAM NORMS AND CONFORMITY

One of the characteristics of small groups noted by Hare (1976) is the development of norms that reflect expectations of behavior on the part of members. Norms provide guidelines for the individual and also serve to indicate the behaviors that can be expected of others (Shaw, 1976). Such standards produce a uniformity of behavior that further serves to identify and maintain the group. Team norms may call for appropriate, nonaggressive behavior on the part of members, for regular attendance at team meetings, for contributing to the work of the team, and for not monopolizing the team discussion with irrelevant material. Norms may cover such diverse matters as dress codes, appropriate language or jargon, and even the seating arrangements in team meetings. Some norms will be discussed and agreed on by the team as a whole. However, often norms are unspoken, and the insensitive team member may be unaware of certain subtle cues used by other team members to control behavior.

Those who deviate from the norms established by the team may face sanctions ranging from being ignored to dismissal. Thus the group uses various forms of pressure to ensure conformity on the part of its members. Teams of course, develop additional sanctions (reprimands, firings) within the organizational structure that may be employed against nonconforming members. When norms are well established, the team may work quickly and harmoniously, but over-conformity may tend to stifle new ideas and solutions and reduce team effectiveness.

Hollander (1958) noted the variation in the severity of sanctions imposed on a group deviant. He pointed out that deviation is more easily tolerated in participants who have "earned" the right to deviate (which he calls "idiosyncrasy credits") through previous contributions to the group. Thus high-status members are less likely to be punished for deviation from group norms than are low-status members. Furthermore, some norms demand rigid adherence, while others are more easily bypassed; some norms are accepted by all group members, while others may be opposed by a significant majority (Shaw, 1976).

The role of conformity is particularly important in decision-making groups where the final outcome is hindered by the failure to adequately examine various alternatives. If team members fail to give full consideration to certain possible solutions because of fear of ridicule or disapproval, then team decisions may not be as good as if all alternatives were considered. Several authors (Argyris, 1969; Hackman, 1975; Hackman and Morris, 1975) have noted that "conservative" norms regarding group behavior tend to dominate the group so that interpersonal risks are minimized and deviant behaviors are quickly punished. Such conformity may be dysfunctional for team effectiveness.

Fry, Lech, and Rubin (1974) discuss the importance of team norms since they influence other aspects of team functioning. They discovered that inflexible team norms — such as "doctors are more important than other team members," "conflict is dangerous," and "silence means consent" — may be dysfunctional. They conclude that "The cost of failing to develop norms of flexibility, support and openness of communication is high indeed" (p. 38) since the team is then unable to become self-correcting.

ROLE, STATUS, AND POWER

Another important characteristic of groups is noted by Hare (1976): the development of a set of roles or role expectations regarding each member of the group. Some of the roles that may be assumed by group members include "energizer," "information-seeker," "opinion-giver," "evaluator-critic," and "harmonizer," as identified by Benne and Sheats (1948). As the names suggest, the *energizer* is one who "prods the [team] to action or decision, attempts to stimulate or arouse the group to 'greater' or 'higher quality' activity," while the *harmonizer* "mediates the differences between other members, attempts to reconcile disagreements, relieves tension in conflict situations through jesting or pouring oil on troubled waters" (Benne and Sheats, 1948, p. 44).

Once established, such roles are likely to be self-perpetuating, so that deviations from the expected roles may disturb other members. However, role expectations in interdisciplinary teams are also based on other factors such as professional affiliation and position in the organization. Thus, a physical therapist will be looked to by the team for relevant information regarding the patient's range of motion, and the social worker will be expected to have knowledge regarding the family situation. It is important to distinguish role expectations based on team membership and behavior in team meetings from those based on professional identification.

The prestige or status of an individual member will be influenced by the roles that individual takes. Although members may "earn" status by playing a significant role (such as "harmonizer") in the interaction process, to a certain extent status in the team is likely to reflect the prestige of the individual's profession. Status variables have been shown to have important effects on a number of group processes. For example, studies have indicated that higher status individuals receive more communication, are better liked, and give less irrelevant communication to other members than persons of lower status in the group (Thibaut and Kelley, 1959).

Both role and status also relate to *social power* or the ability to influence other members of the group. External prestige often influences other team members even as concerns problems that are unrelated to the expertise of the high status individual. Thus the nurse may take the advice of the physician very seriously in choosing a new car, even though the doctor's expertise may not extend to that subject. In a study of role relations in mental health teams, Zander, Cohen, and Stotland (1959) found a consistent power structure with psychiatrists at the top and psychologists and social workers subordinate. That such external power relationships might be expected to carry over to decisions *within* the team is implied by the findings of Leff, Raven, and Gunn (1964) indicating that psychiatrists tend to be more influenced by other psychiatrists than by psychologists, whereas psychologists appeared to be equally influenced by both.

In a study of the effects of power in groups of mental hygiene workers (Hurwitz, Zander, and Hymovitch, 1968) it was found that high power members communicated more often than low power members, were better liked, and received more communication from both high and lower power members. The authors suggest that low power members experience uneasiness in their interaction with highs and react in an ego defensive manner in the group situation. Such reactions are likely to affect not only team maintenance variables, but also the actual decisions reached by the team. This is because the opinions of high power individuals are likely to be given greater weight regardless of the accuracy of their judgments.

The power of the team member may be based on one or more of several possible sources: French and Raven (1959) have identified five bases of power in small groups. *Reward* power and *coercive* power are related to the subject's perception that the individual has the ability to mediate rewards or punishments. These rewards and punishments might be verbal (such as praise or criticism) or more tangible (such as a promotion or a salary increase). *Legitimate power* is based on the internalized cultural values, acceptance of the social structure, and/or designation by a legitimizing agent. Thus a physician has a legitimate right to prescribe medicine, and the principal of a school has a legitimate right to enforce certain regulations. *Referent power* is based on the subject's identification with a power-holder, as when the boss' secretary attains power because of her association with a powerful figure. Finally, *expert power* refers to the subject's perception that the power-holder has special knowledge or expertise. Consultants are often awarded power on the basis of their expertise. All five bases of power will have some relevance for the interaction and outcomes of the team and may be related to the choice of team leader.

THE TEAM LEADER

Leadership has long been thought of as a personal trait, a collection of skills possessed by individuals to a greater or lesser degree, a continuum along which individuals might be ordered according to how much of the trait they possessed. However, more recent concepts (Gibb, 1969; Steiner, 1972) have tended to focus on leadership behavior rather than leadership traits. In reviewing previous attempts at definition of the group leader, several approaches have been noted (Gibb, 1969; Carter, 1953). The leader has been variously identified as the individual who holds a particular office ("chairman" or "president"), one who helps the group move toward its goals, one who is identified by other group members, one who has influence over others, one who is the focus of group behaviors, or one who engages in leadership behaviors.

Although the leader may emerge spontaneously from the interaction of a team, in most cases team leadership is awarded by the parent organization. Thus a physical therapist is asked to coordinate a rehabilitation team, or a psychiatrist is asked to head up a mental health team. However, unless the team members accept the legitimacy of the designated leader, she or he may not be able to fulfill the functions of team leader. Since frequently the individual so designated does in fact already wield considerable influence over group members, that individual is usually accepted to some extent as a team leader.

Regardless of whether a leader has previously been assigned by the organization, it is possible for one or more leaders to emerge during the interactions of the team. Leadership functions may be concentrated primarily in one team member or may be distributed across a number of members. In some teams, leadership roles may shift as the task progresses, so that individuals with differing skills may exert more influence during various phases of the team's activities.

In an analysis of the primary health care team, Parker (1972) identified five aspects of "team leadership": patient coordination and management, team management, charismatic or spiritual leadership, primary patient relationship, and medical decision making. These roles need not all be filled by the same individual and some may shift from one team member to another. While some, such as medical decision making, are directly related to the responsibilities and competencies of the physician, other leadership roles can be filled by any team member.

Since the leadership functions that have been identified cover a broad range of activities and behaviors, it is unlikely that they could all be carried out by only one member of the team. Krech and Crutchfield (1948), for example, have indicated 14 functions that might be performed by a group leader: the leader is seen as executive, planner, policymaker, expert, external group representative, controller of internal relationships, purveyor of rewards and punishments, arbitrator, exemplar, group symbol, surrogate for individual responsibility, ideologist, father figure, or scapegoat. As Cartwright and Zander (1968) have pointed out, "It becomes evident that one person could seldom be effectively responsible for them all" (p. 305). Thus various members of the team may share these functions, assuming those that are ascribed to them by other team members or for which their behavior is most suited.

A distinction is frequently made between a "task leader" and a "social-emotional leader" (Bales and Slater, 1955). The task leader assumes those functions of coordination and planning necessary for task performance, while the social-emotional leader is responsible for team maintenance activities, often serving as a mediator and calming force for the group. Cartwright and Zander

(1968) discuss the two major categories of group functions, "goal achievement" and "group maintenance," pointing out that while one leader may perform both types of functions, in some situations task-oriented or social-emotional "specialists" may be required for effective group performance. For example, although the physician may have been assigned responsibility for coordination of task-directed activities, the social worker may maintain team interaction by mediating disputes, encouraging and motivating the other team members, and relieving team tensions. The social-emotional leader is often better liked by the group than the task leader, but the latter may be more respected. The overall effectiveness of the team will be determined in part by the interaction of these leaders. Competition between them can be quite disruptive to the team, while agreement on significant goals and cooperation in methods of approach can facilitate both goal achievement and team maintenance.

When only one team leader emerges, that leader must demonstrate skills in dealing with both task-oriented and social-emotional functions. Which functions are most essential is likely to vary with the nature of the task, the characteristics of the team, and other variables. Fiedler (1968), for example, has demonstrated that a leader primarily concerned with task completion is likely to be most effective when the situation is one defined as either very easy or very hard, while the more interpersonally oriented leader is more successful when the situation is of intermediate difficulty.

Interestingly, Fiedler concludes that since the effectiveness of the group depends on how the leader's style fits the specific situation at hand, and since most people will be effective leaders in certain situations and not in others, more effort should be given to changing the group situation to fit the leader rather than attempting to change the leader's personality and leadership style to match the situation. Fiedler offers several specific suggestions for changing the group situation. For example, the leader's power can be changed (by increasing or decreasing his authority), or changes can be made in the structure of the task or in the composition of the group.

On the other hand, Shaw (1976) suggests that the leader may be able to vary his or her style with the favorableness of the situation, becoming more responsive to social-emotional factors in moderately difficult group situations, and more directive as the situation becomes extremely favorable or unfavorable. He notes that "The group leader often errs in this respect especially when the group-task situation becomes highly unfavorable. Empirical evidence suggests that he should become more directive, whereas all too often he becomes less directive in his interactions with other members of the group" (p. 395).

The applicability of these concepts to the interdisciplinary team has yet to be empirically demonstrated, and the area is in need of further investigation.

TEAM INTERACTION

Among the group characteristics noted by Hare (1976) were the development of a *network of interpersonal attraction* and the *interaction* of group members. Positive and negative feelings for each other often become the focus of attention in therapeutic groups. However, in teams such feelings may be ignored in the face of more immediate task demands. Yet affective reactions to other members can exert a powerful force in almost any kind of group, and although team membership may offer more tangible rewards (such as promotions, salary increases, and professional status), the approval of other team members may be the strongest and most immediate payoff for teamwork.

Initially team members enter a new group clothed in the professional "position" they hold in the organizational setting. Each position is associated with certain role expectations, status values, and "rights and privileges" — all this quite apart from the individual who occupies that position. Similarly, there are certain built-in relationships between professions that will affect interactions. For example, the role expectations of a doctor and a nurse, a psychiatrist and a social worker, or a teacher and a psychologist will to a considerable extent structure these relationships regardless of how the individuals regard one another. Yet, while professional positions will affect the amount and type of interaction between those individuals who fill them, attractions and antagonisms are often reactions to *people* rather than to job titles. It may be that the personal characteristics of the team member most strongly affect his interactions with others in the group.

Interpersonal attraction has been related to physical attractiveness, similarity of attitudes and beliefs, and compatibility of needs (Shaw, 1976), and it is likely that such factors also affect patterns of attraction and antagonism within the team. Even professionals are more likely to like those who have beliefs, attitudes, and ideas similar to their own. Sociometric techniques can be used to measure these patterns by asking participants to rank all the members along some dimension, or identify members of the group with whom they would or would not like to work, or members they like best.

The network of interpersonal attraction within a team may represent a unique configuration that is an important aspect of the group's identity. In addition, these patterns of interpersonal relations (along with the interprofessional perceptions explored earlier), play a major role in determining the productivity of the team.

COMPOSITION OF THE TEAM

The effectiveness of any team is to a great extent a function of the individuals who comprise its membership. As Shaw (1976) has suggested, age, sex, and other personal attributes of group participants are important because they affect the behavior of the individual, the reaction of other members to that individual, and the overall composition of the group. An important element in the group's composition and ultimate effectiveness is the homogeneity of the group with regard to these individual characteristics.

In discussing the difficulties in assessing the effects of group composition on productivity, Steiner (1972) has observed:

> Heterogeneity with respect to a given attribute may augment potential productivity but greatly increase the complexity of the process which must occur in order for the group to realize its full potential. Thus, for example, a group whose members each possess unique information concerning a topic may have the potential to produce a high quality judgment because their total available information is very great. Such a group is likely to experience greater difficulty in evaluating and pooling information than a group with more homogeneous members'' (p. 197).

Since an interdisciplinary team is by definition a heterogeneous group, we may expect, according to Steiner, some difficulty in integrating information. Hopefully, this will be offset by more effective outcomes because of the diversity of the information available to the group.

The composition of teams may vary in a number of ways. Let us briefly examine some of those factors and note how they may affect team functioning.

Profession

In most cases, the team will be professionally heterogeneous, with a number of disciplines and specialities represented. However, teams may be composed primarily of closely-related professions, such as dentists and dental hygienists. As indicated above, teams composed of professionals of varied skills and expertise will have more total information available in their deliberations than a group with more limited, overlapping, and perhaps even redundant information, but the heterogeneous group may experience greater difficulty in assimilating and integrating such diverse data. Although the potential quality of judgment may be much higher in a heterogeneous grouping, the complexity introduced by those differences may prove counter-productive.

Additionally, Steiner notes, "Probably heterogeneity is also more likely than homogeneity to promote antagonisms among members" (Steiner, 1972, p. 107). Since professionals of varied disciplines, experience, and training will view the client in terms of a frame of reference or theoretical model drawn from that training, the more heterogeneous the team members, the more varied their ways of approaching the client's problems. Even the language or professional jargon of the various disciplines may lead to confusion and misunderstandings. Such antagonisms may divert attention from the task of decision making, introducing considerable static in the process and reducing the effectiveness of the team.

Sex

The effect that the sexual composition of the team has upon the group processes is somewhat uncertain. Most teams are mixed groups with a fair proportion of male and female members; however, occasionally all male or all female groups are found in professional settings. The most striking effect may be found in teams where the great majority is of one sex and only one or two representatives of the opposite sex are present. This situation seems to make all participants more aware of sex roles and may tend to give greater or lesser weight to the input of the minority participants. Thus, the opinions of a sole male participant may have greater influence on the team's deliberations than would his contribution if he were merely one of several male participants. In the same way, a sole female member may be reluctant to appear too "aggressive" in an all male team.

Just as heterogeneity along other dimensions, such as professional background, introduces greater complexity into team dynamics, a mixture of male and female team members also seems to complicate interactions and opens up new sources of influence. Results of research on small groups have been somewhat conflicting. For example, mixed sex groups have been found to perform more efficiently than all male groups (Hoffman and Maier, 1961) and less efficiently than either all male or all female groups (Clement and Schiereck, 1973). Mixed sex groups have also been found to be more conforming than same sex groups (Reitan and Shaw, 1964). Shaw (1976) suggests that mixed sex groups may be more concerned about socio-emotional factors, while same sex groups may concentrate on task orientation. Another finding suggests that culturally stereotyped sexual roles may result in greater conformity among female participants, while males are expected to respond competitively.

The effects of sexual composition in interdisciplinary teams is also complicated by the relationship between sex and profession. There tends to be a preponderance of female team members in middle status professions such as nursing or occupational therapy, and more males in higher status professions such as medicine. It is often difficult to separate the effects of profession and sex in the operation of teams in human service settings.

Age

Predictably the age of the team members will have some effect on the processes and outcomes of the group interaction. As with stereotyped sexual roles, cultural expectations related to age can affect the perceptions of team members and increase or decrease the weight given to an individual's opinion. A young physician may be treated differently than an older one. Since age is also likely to be confounded with professional experience and status, it may be difficult to isolate the effects of age alone. It should be noted, however, that since the groups under consideration here are composed primarily of professionals the age span is somewhat reduced. Most of the research dealing with age and group effectiveness has involved children and is not applicable to teams. It may well be that compared to other factors such as ability and experience, age is a relatively less important variable in interdisciplinary teams.

Other Factors

Other personal attributes such as intelligence, dominance, authoritarianism, social sensitivity, and special skills or abilities are also likely to affect the individual's contribution to the team activities. The unique constellation of attributes, abilities, and experience found in each team will determine to a great extent how the team operates and its effectiveness in carrying out its tasks. Results of several studies have suggested that differences in abilities and personality profiles within the group are more conducive to effective problem solving than is group homogeneity (Goldman, 1965; Laughlin, et al., 1969; Hoffman, 1959; Hoffman and Maier, 1961).

In summarizing a review of research on the effects of group composition, Shaw (1976) concludes:

> We have just begun the analysis of group composition effects. It is already clear that such efforts are far more complex than they appeared to be initially. We may hazard a guess that interpersonal compatibility is the basic variable in group composition; the large task facing group dynamics is the theoretical analysis of interpersonal relations so that the compatibility-incompatibility of individual characteristics can be identified (p. 236).

COMMUNICATION NETWORKS

Communication between team members — that is, *who talks to whom* — is a central variable in team interaction. A good deal of research has focused on the determinants and consequences of communication networks in small group functioning. A communication network has been defined as "the arrangement (or pattern) of communication channels among the members of a group" (Shaw, 1976, p. 445). In an attempt to determine the effects of different communication networks on group performance, Bavelas (1948) developed a technique that has been used by a number of other investigators. In this design, subjects are placed alone in cubicles with connecting slots through which messages may be passed. By varying the available slots participants can use, the channels of communication can be controlled by the experimenter. If all slots are open, each participant can communicate with every other participant (termed a completely connected or *comcon* network). Other network designs such as wheels, chains, and circles can be formed by closing designated channels. Experiments in varying communication networks along with variations in the task involved, the number of participants, and other significant factors, have been performed to study a number of relationships involving communication patterns.

One of the significant notions emerging from these studies is that of *centrality* of one's position in the network. Centrality has been defined and measured in a number of ways; however, the concept can best be illustrated by an example (Cartwright and Zander, 1968). In a five-person group arranged in a row (A-B-C-D-E), C holds the most central position (with the shortest total communication distance to every other member), while A and E are in the most peripheral locations. In a circle network where all members are equidistant, all positions are equally central. The importance of the idea lies in the relationship that has been found between centrality and leadership: the individual holding the central position is most likely to emerge as the identified group leader (Shaw, 1976). Furthermore, centrality of position is also related to satisfaction; those members who have more channels of communication available indicate greater satisfaction than those with limited communication outlets. This finding has implications for team morale, since networks that provide only limited communication for a large number of members may suffer morale problems. One way to explain the relationship between satisfaction and centrality is that greater centrality leads to greater feelings of independence, autonomy, and power, thus producing a sense of satisfaction with one's position in the group (Cartwright and Zander, 1968).

Within the limitations of the network, various informal communication structures arise for purposes of exchanging information necessary to complete the task. Two basic organization patterns have been identified: the each-to-all pattern and the centralized organization (Shaw, 1976). In the centralized pattern, all of the data is channeled to one individual who solves the problem and communicates this solution to the other members. This approach is used by some health care and human service teams. The each-to-all pattern involves sharing all information with all participants, who then solve the problem independently.

The particular communication network used by the group usually determines the type of organizational structure that emerges. Centralized networks usually lead to centralized organizations, while networks that do not place any member in a centralized position are likely to develop as each-to-all organizations (Shaw, 1976). Shaw also points out that centralized communication networks appear to be more effective with simple problems, while complex problems are more efficiently handled in decentralized networks.

It is difficult to generalize from these laboratory studies to the interdisciplinary team, but some parallels do come to mind. Some teams appear to have clear-cut, almost rigid communication channels with a leader who controls and directs the discussion to an unusual degree. In such cases, the leader may direct questions to other team members and receive answers from them in turn, but there may be little or no communication between team members themselves. Such an extreme situation would clearly represent the centralized network and centralized organization. In contrast, in the decentralized pattern all members communicate freely with all other members, and each participant has access to the total available information.

Many authors who are concerned with the effectiveness of the interdisciplinary team emphasize the importance of open communication channels between team members (Rubin and Beckhard, 1972; Haselkorn, 1958; Nagi, 1975; Lacks, Landsbaum, and Stern, 1970). Wagner (1977) points out that Shaw's (1964) findings (that groups with more communication channels perform best on complex tasks while groups with fewer channels are better with simple tasks) suggest that "all-channel" networks may be most effective for the "complex human relations problems" dealt with by the team, as compared with the "wheel" network used by the individual practitioner.

Rubin and Beckhard (1972) indicate that since each team member is a resource, there must be open channels of communication to all other members. Haselkorn considers communication a crucial element in interprofessional collaboration and examines some of the problems that may interfere with communication. Lacks, Landsbaum, and Stern (1970) developed a training laboratory experience to increase communication in a children's psychiatric team as a way of improving team performance.

We will examine some other aspects of team communication in Chapter Ten. The interested reader can find a further discussion of communication among team members in Horwitz (1970). The two literature reviews by Tichy — one covering literature on teams (1974), the other dealing with relevant behavioral science research (1975) — are also pertinent to this topic.

TEAM COHESIVENESS

Another important element in team interaction is the cohesiveness of the team. Although cohesiveness has been defined in a number of ways, most would agree with Cartwright's statement (1968, p. 91) that it "refers to the degree to which the members of the group desire to remain in the group." Interpersonal attraction among group members has often been used as a measure of group cohesiveness, since attraction to other members appears to be an important component of an individual's attraction to and desire to remain in the group. Cohesiveness is regarded in some ways as the "glue" that holds the group together. The more cohesive the team, the higher the likelihood it will maintain itself over a period of time and exert influence over its members. Thus cohesiveness is an important factor in determining the willingness of team members to contribute to the work of the team and thus to its outcomes.

Earlier we indicated that several factors found to be related to interpersonal attraction may also be important in determining group cohesiveness. Certainly, groups whose members are attracted to one another by common interests and attitudes, compatible needs, and other shared characteristics seem more likely to "stick together." However, other factors may also affect the cohesiveness of teams. Thibaut and Kelley (1959) have pointed out that a participant's attraction to the group depends on the relative costs and rewards that group membership will bring. Most people have had many group experiences in the past, and these experiences form a standard of *comparison* against which present or future groups can be compared. According to Thibaut and Kelley, the more one's expectations of the outcomes of membership exceed the individual's *comparison level*, the more one will be attracted to that group. An individual may be drawn to a team because of its goals, its activities, the kind of leadership demonstrated, or other incentives. Cartwright's article (1968) indicated that the *motives* of the potential group member are also important. These include the need for affiliation, prestige, recognition, or other rewards the group may offer.

Thus, according to Cartwright, cohesiveness depends on four sets of interacting variables: the *needs* of the participants, the *incentives* offered, the *expectations* of the members about the outcomes, and the *comparison levels* held by group members. Even in situations where team membership is a mandatory "part of the job" rather than a voluntary elective, these factors are likely to be important in determining whether members feel they are an integral part of a team or simply going through the motions.

COALITIONS

Along with the factors that tend to bring teams together into cohesive units are a number of factors that lead to divisions and conflicts. Ideally, teams are cooperative ventures in which members pool their individual resources in order to arrive at a better outcome. Thus members of a mental health team will pool their talents, professional training, experience, and the information they have gathered about a client, in order to make a diagnosis, predict the client's future behavior, establish a treatment plan, or carry out the treatment. Such an endeavor is assumed to produce an outcome beneficial to the client and to team members as well.

However, as we have seen in our discussion of team cohesiveness, individual prestige, recognition from other members, a promotion, or salary increase may also be considered incentives for some team members. Thus, as in most group situations, competitiveness can affect the actions of team members, and most teams are likely to contain elements of both cooperation and competitiveness. In the parlance of game theory, such teams are said to be engaged in mixed-motive games.

The sociometric techniques used to study interpersonal attraction within groups often reveal a number of subgroups within the larger unit. These smaller groups, held together by friendship or mutual liking, are generally referred to as cliques. Although cliques may affect communication patterns within a team, they will not necessarily affect the outcome or decisions made by the team as a whole. When a subgroup is drawn together to affect outcomes, the term *coalition* is used. For example, a clique may decide to work together against another individual or subgroup within the larger group, and in this case a coalition would emerge.

Most of the work on coalition formation has taken place in laboratory settings with individuals who are initially strangers. These studies generally do not operate long enough or in such a way as to reveal the role of interpersonal attraction in coalition formation (Carlins and Raven, 1969). Research on coalitions often makes use of triads, in which two members join together in opposition to a third person in order to control the outcomes of the group.

Several theories of coalition formation have been suggested, and these have tended to focus on how coalitions form in relation to the resources available to each potential participant. For example, the minimum resource theory (Gamson, 1961) contends that coalitions are likely to form between persons who control the minimum resources necessary to control the outcome. Thus if A has five points, with B and C each having three points, a coalition would most likely occur between B and C. Although some attention has been given to the role of additional factors such as interpersonal relations, most research in this area has attempted to control for such variables rather than investigate them.

The complexities of coalition formation in natural group settings remain generally unexplained. Since the participants may be seeking any number of possible rewards in addition to the expressed purpose and expected outcomes of the team conference, we might expect that coalition formation would be highly unpredictable. Gamson (1961) refers to this lack of predictability as the "utter confusion theory," reflecting the lack of understanding of the variables determining coalitions.

Despite our frequent inability to understand or predict the specific coalitions that may emerge in many human service teams, they can be a significant factor in determining outcomes. Using a mental health team as an example, we can visualize a number of ways in which coalitions might operate. Sometimes coalitions seem to form around professional identification — with psychiatrists, psychologists, social workers, or other professional groups uniting along professional lines to oppose recommendations made by other group members or other coalitions. Often two or more professional groups join against a third, as when the psychiatrists and social workers in the team unite to oppose the opinions of the psychologist(s). Ideological or theoretical values can also lead to the formation of coalitions. For instance, team members with a psychoanalytic bent may join together in opposing a treatment plan based on techniques of behavior modification, or two or three therapists with primary interest and expertise in individual treatment may rigorously oppose a recommendation of group counseling for a client.

Coalitions may be seen as both indicative of and contributing to the potential conflict and divisiveness within a team. Coalitions may be subtle and more or less "under the table," or may be clearly recognized by the group. They may be relatively permanent (with members of the coalition consistently supporting the position of other coalition partners, with an implicit understanding that they will in turn be supported), or unstable and changing (with considerable switching of coalition membership as issues change). It would appear that the more stable the team, the more likely the formation of clearcut coalition subgroups. It should be noted, however, that sometimes when a particular coalition exerts excessive power over group decisions, there is a corresponding loss of morale among other members who may feel that their input is not valued. Thus the rewards offered them by group membership are considerably diminished, and cohesiveness may be reduced to the point where team effectiveness is seriously threatened and/or the group may disintegrate. In other cases where a powerful coalition threatens the functioning of the team, new coalitions may be formed to counteract this threat. Individuals who may oppose each other on ideological or other grounds may unite against a common threat, at least on significant issues. This continuous realignment of team participants in various subgroups makes it difficult to predict the direction of coalition formation in natural groupings outside the laboratory situation.

OTHER FACTORS

There are a number of other factors that may set limits or in some way structure the interaction of team members. These include the size of the team, the physical environment in which it meets, how often it meets and for how long, and its degree of formality.

Size of the Team

Much attention has been given to the question of an optimal size for decision-making groups, but results are not clearcut since size interacts with a number of other variables. A task that is divisible and can be shared by individual team members working alone or in smaller units will require enough participants to adequately complete each task component. In these cases, then, the optimal size relates directly to the number of task components. In the interdisciplinary team, optimal size may be dependent on the number of specialists required by a particular case or by the requirements of a hospital ward or unit.

As a team increases in size, the number of possible relationships between members increases rapidly. For example, in a 3-member group there are 3 possible relationships, but in a 6-member group there are 15 possible paired relationships. It has been pointed out that while a larger group has more resources available for meeting task demands, the individual contribution of each member is reduced as group size increases and only the more forceful members can make their opinions known (Hare, 1976).

Physical Environment

The physical setting in which the team interacts may affect its operation in several ways. A light airy room with comfortable seating arrangements, adequate lighting, and good temperature control will allow team participants to concentrate on the tasks at hand rather than be preoccupied with their own feelings of discomfort. A room that is too hot or too cold or has uncomfortable chairs may serve to unduly prolong (or shorten) the meeting.

The seating arrangement both shapes and is molded by the interaction of the members. As a particular team develops a mode of interaction, it will spontaneously modify the arrangement of chairs to fit its style of operation. A formal arrangement generally denotes a more constrained interaction. In any case, no matter what arrangement is adopted, often one or two individuals will place their chairs in an idiosyncratic position not in keeping with the total arrangement.

The physical setting may affect the performance of the team in more specific ways. Research has indicated that seating arrangements may affect the flow of communication and the quality of the group interaction, and that "when members of a group are seated at a round table, there is a strong tendency for members to communicate with persons across the table and facing them rather than with persons adjacent to them" (Shaw, 1976, pp. 133-134).

Although the relationship between status and seating is not clearcut, evidence suggests that seating arrangements play a role in leadership selection where leaders have not already been assigned. Positions at the head of the table or in the most central location are generally regarded as having higher status than more peripheral positions. Students, particularly in medical settings, often comment on the relationship between professional status and seat location in team meetings. Frequently physicians sit together at the center of the group, with psychologists and social workers adjacent, and nurses, physical and occupational therapists, and other professionals seated at varying distances from the center.

Territoriality with regard to seating has also been noted. In cases where seats are not formally assigned, participants will frequently establish territorial rights to a particular chair in a certain location, and return to that seat each meeting. New members are expected to take seats that do not "belong" to anyone else and may be resented if they unknowingly usurp another member's chair.

Formality-Informality of the Team

One of the dimensions along which teams may vary markedly is the formality or informality of their procedures. The two hypothetical teams described in Chapter Six varied greatly in terms of formality, the medical team conference showing a much more formal procedure than the mental health team conference. The degree of formality in a team meeting is apparent in the physical arrangement of the seating. Seats lined up in neat rows reminiscent of a formal classroom suggest a communication network and style of interaction quite different from that suggested by a casual, even somewhat sloppy circle of chairs. Seating is only one rather obvious aspect of formality. More crucial to the eventual outcomes of the team is the formality of the group interaction itself. A casual and relaxed atmosphere may lead to more spontaneous and more frequent comments by the participants, while in a more formal context the interaction may be somewhat stilted and reserved. On the other hand, greater informality may encourage more irrelevant information and lead to a less effective use of the time and energy of the team members.

Length and Frequency of Team Meetings

The professionals who make up teams are faced with heavy demands on their time. Often they are members of several teams, committees, and other decision-making groups. Team sessions may last anywhere from a half-hour to a half-day, or in some rare instances even a full day. The effects of duration on the group process is mixed. In therapy groups or self-awareness groups the purpose of the session may be to move from cognitive to more affective expression, and here increased duration even to the point of marathon sessions may be quite conducive to meeting group goals. However, in teams that make decisions critical to the future of an individual, shorter sessions appear to be more effective.

It seems likely that the relationship between duration and effectiveness may be represented by an inverted U-shaped function, with both very short and very long sessions proving less effective than sessions of moderate length. Short sessions do not give the group an opportunity to share the information that needs to be shared and integrate it in a meaningful way. Long sessions tend to be tiring, and participants sometimes become less involved and more careless in their judgments as the session progresses. Team members who become anxious to leave may agree to courses of action that they might otherwise oppose. Individuals have different levels of tolerance for long sessions, and those who have the stamina to sustain their position may find that their input gains weight as the conference continues and other members begin to tire.

Team meetings may be held once a day, once a week, once a month, or even less frequently. Sessions may be scheduled regularly or called when a decision is pending or a problem arises. The frequency with which the team meets is related to the interaction between team members. Teams that meet infrequently may not develop a high degree of cohesiveness. On the other hand, too frequent meetings can be resented by busy professionals who may lose interest in the team, decrease their involvement, and thus reduce their input. With frequent sessions, potential antagonisms between members are more likely to surface, and this too may reduce productivity.

Stability

Some teams are highly stable, with a fixed group of participants meeting frequently over a long period of time. Unstable teams are those whose membership frequently shifts, with different members attending each session. There is little continuity or cohesiveness in an unstable group, and much less opportunity to develop shared perceptions and a shared language. The rules by which decisions are made may change markedly from session to session, depending on who is in attendance. If the group is too unstable, it may not meet the criteria for a team spelled out in Chapter One.

At the other extreme are those teams that have interacted so closely and for so long that the individual team members have come to perceive and respond to events in a very similar manner. Certain situations seem to demand this kind of consensus, so a great deal of effort is sometimes devoted to developing a common framework. For example, when a behavior modification procedure or token economy system is introduced in an agency, there must be agreement among the staff as to the behavior that will be rewarded. This agreement is difficult to achieve if there is rapid turnover in the team or if members attend irregularly.

TEAM DECISION MAKING

In Chapter Six we examined the decision-making process as a major activity of the team. At that time we looked at the decision process generally and at some of the underlying concepts. In this section we are interested in how the dynamics of the team have impact on those decisions. That is, are decisions reached through team discussion and a sharing of information different in some systematic way from decisions reached by individual professionals acting alone?

The Risky Shift in Decision Making

Earlier in this chapter, we discussed evidence that group norms tend to be rather conservative and that group conformity may serve to stifle originality and creative contributions by team members. In contrast to this generally accepted view is the interesting paradox of what has been termed the "risky-shift" phenomenon in group decision making. Findings suggest that in certain situations decisions reached by groups may in fact reflect a greater willingness to take risks than those reached by individuals working alone.

This finding was first demonstrated by Stoner (1961) who studied male graduate students in industrial management. Each subject was first asked to independently (and privately) indicate the level of risk he would be willing to accept for a series of life dilemma problems. For example, an individual is offered a job with a new company. The job has an uncertain future, but offers higher pay and the possibility of a partnership if the company survives. The present job offers lifetime security and a good pension, but a modest salary. The subject is required to indicate the lowest probability of the company's succeeding that would make a move worthwhile (e.g., 1 in 10, 5 in 10, etc.). The group then discussed each problem until a decision was reached regarding the degree of risk acceptable to the group. Instead of showing a decrease in risk taking as might be expected from studies in group conformity, the group decisions were *riskier* than the average of the individual decisions.

The original experiment has been replicated frequently in order to verify these findings and attempt to explain them. The risky shift has been demonstrated with a variety of subjects and tasks, and several hypotheses have been suggested to account for the phenomenon.

Most of the studies in this area have made use of the *choice-dilemma question-n aire* (Kogan and Wallach, 1964) that contained 12 real-life dilemmas similar to the example above. In each case, an individual is faced with a safe alternative with a lower payoff or a riskier choice with the potential of greater gain, and the subject must select the degree of risk which he or she views as acceptable. Other studies have used problem-solving tasks (with subjects choosing the level of difficulty of items they wish to attempt as a measure of risk taking) and gambling situations.

What are the significant factors in the group that cause individuals to shift their decision? This question has stimulated a great deal of research. Most of the studies have involved group discussion until consensus was reached. Although it was earlier thought that establishing consensus might be the critical factor, Wallach and Kogan (1965) demonstrated that the shift could occur with discussion alone but not with consensus alone. On the other hand, "information exchange" without discussion has also lead to a risky shift (Teger and Pruitt, 1967; Blank, 1968).

In an extensive review of the literature on the risky-shift phenomenon (Dion, Baron, & Miller, 1970) four major explanations were identified: diffusion of responsibility, persuasion, familiarization, and the cultural value hypothesis. We will briefly examine these explanations, since they have some bearing on how teams reach decisions about their client.

Diffusion of Responsibility Hypothesis

Stated in its simplest terms, this hypothesis suggests that a risk-taking situation may induce anxiety or fear of failure in subjects and that the sharing of responsibility with the group reduces these fears and allows for a greater degree of risk. Although some research (Wallach, Kogan, & Bem, 1964) provided support for such an explanation, other studies (Marquis, 1962; Pruitt and Teger, 1969) have raised some questions. In further modification and elaboration of the responsibility-diffusion notion, it has been suggested that the diffusion may be based on affective bonds developed between group members during group discussion. In a study (Dion, Miller, & Magnon, 1970) conducted in response to certain methodological problems encountered in previous attempts to examine the affective bond idea, group cohesiveness was experimentally manipulated to produce a group high in cohesiveness and another low in cohesiveness. Contrary to expectations, the highly cohesive group showed less risky shift than the group low in cohesiveness. However, the researchers offer an interesting interpretation of these results, in that ''as group members become more attracted to one another they also become more loath to minimize *personal* responsibility or displace responsibility for failure onto their fellow group members'' (Dion, Baron, & Miller, 1970, p. 320). Such a possibility would have real implications for the operation of a shift toward greater risk in ongoing teams in which cohesiveness had developed. In view of the contradictory evidence around the responsibility-diffusion hypothesis, some researchers have turned to other possible explanations.

Persuasion Hypothesis

What Dion, et al. (1970) have called the ''persuasion'' hypothesis holds that high risk takers are more influential and persuasive in the group, and thus the shift of the group toward greater risk is in reaction to this leadership. In support of this theory, several studies have found a relationship between the initial risk allowed by individuals and the influence on group discussion attributed to them by group members in post-session ratings (Wallach, Kogan, & Burt, 1965). However, it has been pointed out (Kelley and Thibaut, 1969; Shaw, 1976) that the parallel between the shift in the group and the opinion of the high risk takers may be an artifact of the situation. If the group shifts toward greater risk, it will *appear* as though they are shifting toward the opinion of those who initially held this position. Even when it is demonstrated that the group members *perceive* high risk-takers to be more influential, this may only reflect an assumption on their part that since the group has shifted toward higher risk, the high-risk takers *must* have been influential. There have been attempts to pursue this further by examining personality differences of initially high and low risk-takers. But as Dion, et al. suggest, there is a need for more direct evidence, based on observation of the group process with independent evaluation of the relative influence of various group members.

Familiarization Hypothesis

Most researchers who have dealt with the risky-shift phenomenon have seen it as a group effect and have looked for explanations in terms of "What does the group do to change the risk taking of individuals?" However, a few (Bateson, 1966; Flanders and Thistlethwaite, 1967) have sought an explanation in terms of individual rather than group processes. The familiarization hypothesis suggests that what is important in the risk-taking experimental paradigm is the greater familiarity with the problems presented. This presumably leads to a concomitant reduction in uncertainty and an increased willingness to take risks. In the usual risky-shift experiment, group discussion serves to increase familiarity with the pros and cons of each specific alternative, and it is the additional experience or understanding of the item rather than the group process per se that leads to a shift in risk. Although initial studies by Bateson (1966) and by Flanders and Thistlethwaite (1967) demonstrated a shift to greater risk following familiarization alone (without group discussion), later studies have failed to replicate these findings (Ferguson and Vidmar, 1970; Myers, 1967; and Pruitt and Teger, 1967). Thus familiarization does not seem to offer a clear and sufficient explanation for the risky-shift phenomenon (Dion, et al., 1970).

Cultural Value Hypothesis

As reviewed and summarized by Dion, Baron, and Miller (1970), Brown's (1965) theory of risk taking assumes that cultural values encourage risk taking under some conditions and caution under others, and that a risky-shift would occur in those situations in which risk is supported by cultural values. Under such conditions the risk value would serve to direct the group discussion so that individuals could gain relevant information about the decision and about the position of other group members. The discussion would not only give the individual additional support for risk taking but also reveal the degree of risk others are willing to take, thereby encouraging the individual to move in a more risky direction. Experimental results seem generally supportive of this explanation, but contradictory findings have also been reported.

Summary

In summarizing research on the risky-shift, Dion, et al. (1970) conclude that although at the present time the cultural value hypothesis offers the strongest single explanation, "when we reach a complete understanding of group decision-making and risk-taking, it should not surprise us if propositions from several competing theoretical positions turn out to be true" (p. 370). The authors further point out that up to now very little attention has been given to such phenomena in "real" groups. "Real" groups may differ in several ways from those used for experimental purposes, including differences in status and in the consequences of the decision.

For example, group members brought together in a research study have not had the previous experience with each other that team members have had, they do not have the status differences that exist in teams, and they are usually dealing with hypothetical problems rather than with decisions that will have real impact on the group or other individuals.

The data concerning the riskiness of group decisions does have implications for group decision making in other contexts, however. First, it puts into a different perspective the information regarding conformity pressures in groups and suggests that while groups may sometimes come to more conservative decisions, this is not *necessarily* the case.

More recent research (Myers and Lamm, 1976) has suggested that "risky-shift" may have been a misnomer, since the shift may be toward either greater or lesser risk. Thus the term "group polarization" has been used to refer to changes in group responses as a result of group discussion (in jury decisions, ethical decisions, and other choice situations) in addition to risk taking. Second, as Dion, et al. (1970) indicate, research on the shift-to-risk has also shown that the decisions of the group may at times be less rational and less responsible than individual decisions (Bem, et al., 1965). Such findings are important in examining the effectiveness of group decision making in the human service professions.

One study reported by Winter (1976) applied findings from the risky-shift literature to the team approach. Using college students as subjects, Winter found that willingness to provide rehabilitation services to hypothetical clients who could be regarded as "high risk" was greater among groups than among individuals, and that persuasion may have been a factor in the shift to risk. Winter concluded that "a team approach used in making decisions about acceptance or rejection of applicants for rehabilitation services may provide the impetus for more acceptant and liberal views about clients and may thus provide for more extensive delivery of rehabilitation services to individuals with severe conditions" (p.580).

Wagner (1977) reported on an earlier study in which he had examined teamwork performance in terms of service plans made by teams and by individual practitioners. A major conclusion was that "team service plans are more holistic and that team practitioners, when compared with nominal groups of independent practitioners, expressed more of a need to become involved in the totality of the client's life" (Wagner, 1977, p. 213). In addition, he found teams to more frequently consider input of several professions and be concerned with the client's "significant others," while individual practitioners developed more specific recommendations and more unique service plans. These findings suggest that team decision making may indeed lead to different outcomes than when such decisions are made by professionals acting alone.

Some authors express concern about the results of team decision making. While more decision-making responsibilities are being delegated to interdisciplinary teams, in some cases team members may be unclear as to what those responsibilities are. Fenton, Yoshida, Maxwell, and Kaufman (1979) found that many members of interdisciplinary placement teams responsible for decisions concerning the delivery of special education services did not recognize the teams' responsibilities. Rae-Grant and Marcuse (1968) warned that one of the hazards of teamwork is the idea of "shared responsibility": "The myth that the total team is effectively discharging responsibility for a given patient may be the fact that no one fully accepts responsibility or feels himself to be ultimately accountable for what happens" (p. 4). They also point out that some members may see the anonymity of team decision making as an excuse for less responsible behavior. Weiner and Raths (1959) found that team diagnostic and prognostic decisions are not more accurate as a result of the team meeting. They suggest that some of the team's time may be wasted and that other team activities might be more useful.

Nagi (1975) indicated that two major aspects of team decision making are structure and substance. By structure he is referring to the "hierarchical" and "equalitarian" models of decision making in teams and to the constraints imposed on the team by the parent organization. Substance refers to "what agreements and disagreements take place among team members in regard to the substance of the decision" (p. 191). Differences in professional background and other characteristics of individual team members can be expected to lead to certain disagreements. Rubin and Beckhard (1972) stress that such differences can make it difficult to reach consensus on the team's decisions, with the result that team members feel less commitment to those decisions. A recognition that all members may be involved in implementing a decision is one of the major arguments for shared decision making.

Chapter 8

Team Evaluation and Research

"Does the team approach work?" is a question that is often raised and for which we have no answer. In fact, we might argue that the question itself, phrased in such general terms, is almost meaningless. We must have answers to a multitude of narrower, more specific questions about teams and team effectiveness before we can even begin to address such a broad question. It may well be that when we have reached such a point the question itself will seem irrelevant.

Past studies of team effectiveness have left much to be desired. Halstead (1976), after a selective review of 25 years of literature concerning team care in chronic illness, says:

> The conclusions drawn . . . are not particularly reassuring. . . . An avalanche of articles and reports has been published which almost unanimously endorse the proposition that team care is desirable, relevant and effective in many areas of health delivery. Yet the evidence to support these claims is exceedingly slim (pp. 509-510).

Halstead divides the published reports about the team approach into three broad categories: opinion-based articles, descriptive articles, and the "study base" made up of controlled and comparative studies of the team. The third group was far smaller than the first two categories; Halstead summarizes 10 studies that fall into the third category.

Among the conclusions drawn by Halstead are the following:

> On the whole, coordinated team care appears to be more effective than the customary fragmented care currently received by most persons with long-term illnesses. . . .

> Team care research, while presenting special problems, is in fact possible (p. 510).

In this chapter we are concerned with two aspects of the study of teams: evaluation and research. It can be argued that one term subsumes the other. In this instance the division is made on the basis that evaluative studies are concerned with the more short-term goal of direct practical intervention with specific, functioning teams, whereas research studies are more concerned with long-term goals of theory building and theory testing. There is indeed some overlap, which in the long run will prove to be a positive influence: as theory is tested in operational settings, both theory and practice are improved.

THE NEED FOR EVALUATION

A number of parties are concerned with the evaluation of the team approach: the client, the professional who is a member of a team, the organization in which the team operates, and another group often referred to as "third party payers." While we might assume that what is best for the client is best for all concerned, this is not necessarily true, and what may seem to be an unqualified "good" or benefit for one interested group may not be a benefit for others.

For example, although it is socially acceptable to say that what is wanted is the "best" in health care or human services, it is just not true unless qualified by some statement concerning the acceptable *costs* of health care. Therefore, it seems reasonable to evaluate those costs in relation to benefit received by the client.

To look at the need for evaluation from the individual *client's* point of view, we probably must make several assumptions. First among these is that the client's overriding interest is in the benefits that come to him or her as a result of the work of the team. We must be careful to separate individual client benefits from other social benefits of which the client may approve but which do not reflect directly on the client. For example, since the cost of health care is borne only in part by the individual, if the health care team is a more cost effective means of delivering health care but delivers that care at less than maximum quality, then the team approach is of dubious benefit to the individual. It is also assumed that the client values maintaining or enhancing his or her own quality of life. Another assumption is that there are alternative systems for the delivery of health care and that each holds the possibility of greater benefit to the client.

We can also look at the need for evaluation from the point of view of the *professional*. The needs of the professional and the client coincide in some instances and not in others. For example, the professional certainly shares the client's interest in successful treatment (although what constitutes "success" may differ quite a bit between professional and client). However, the "efficient" use of time may be a crucial issue for the professional but much less important to an individual client, even though it benefits all clients if time is used efficiently. Similarly, if the team functions well in educating its members, there are indirect benefits to all clients even if the direct benefits to any particular client are not so apparent. The professional's main interest in the evaluation of team effectiveness may be in whether the team operation enhances the professional's ability to provide better service.

From the perspective of the *organization*, evaluation reflects the desire to assess how well the team is meeting broad organizational goals. While it would seem that such interests mesh with both client interests and professional needs, this may not be the case. The organization may place its main emphasis on how smoothly the team accommodates to or fits in with the organizational structure, and its evaluation may take this thrust. The institution may also share with third party payers a common interest in keeping costs down.

WHAT TO EVALUATE?

There are many aspects of teamwork that can be evaluated: the improvement of the quality of life for the client, the cost effectiveness of the team, or the effectiveness of the team process as an educational medium for team members.

We can return to our general model of the team system shown in Figure 1-1 (Chapter One) and use this to derive a paradigm for the evaluation of the team approach. Each part of the model is important to the evaluation process. If we can determine the goals of the team and relate these goals to activities and outcomes relative to the needs of the client, the professionals, and the organization, then we will have made the first step in team evaluation. Thus the initial component becomes the identification of team goals (both task and maintenance goals) and the collection of data related to the achievement of those goals.

Clear statements of goals are vital to the evaluation process. Sometimes even when goal statements *are* available and an attempt is made to measure performance against these published goals, the evaluator is told, "But those goals do not really reflect what we are trying to do." There is a real need for teams to formulate in the most explicit terms possible both task and maintenance goals, and all members of the team should be fully aware of the goals that will be used in the evaluation process.

Once goals have been clearly identified and stated, it is necessary to decide what indicators of goal achievement are to be used. It is important that the indicators be closely related to the real goals, since the evaluation process tends to make people focus on those aspects of their performance for which they will be held accountable. Care must be taken in the selection of output indicators in order that they not become substitutes for the goals themselves.

For example, some years ago the State University of New York based the annual budget for its various academic departments on the number of students enrolled. Data were collected for the fall term of each year and extrapolated for the remainder of the year. Thus departmental budgets were in large part determined by a measure of the number of students shown to be attending classes during the fall term. Over time it was noticed that in some cases departments were showing fall term enrollments that were much larger than anticipated. Closer examination showed that the departments in question had moved a higher proportion of their required courses and large lecture sections to the fall term, thereby maximizing upon the indicator used, but not enhancing the real outcome since the total output did not change. Similar instances may be found where an "average daily census" or "beds occupied" figure is used as an indicator of productivity for funding purposes.

QUESTIONS ABOUT TEAM EVALUATION

According to Deming (1975), one of the requirements of an effective evaluation system is a "meaningful operational measure of success or of failure . . . of some proposed treatment applied to specified material, under specified conditions" (p. 56). By "materials" Deming is referring to persons, patients, accounts, products, or "anything else." Of course, the treatment we are interested in evaluating is the use of a team. Keeping Deming's requirement in mind, let us look at some specific questions about team evaluation.

1. **How is team "effectiveness" or "success" to be measured?** Establishing the criteria of success or effectiveness encompasses a number of elements. For example, team effectiveness might be measured on the basis of improvement in the condition of clients, more efficient use of professional time, or expressed satisfaction of team members, administrators, or clients. Such measurement may involve the development of objective instruments to measure whatever outcomes are to be examined.

It is possible then, that we might develop several different criteria of effectiveness and that these criteria may produce contradictory results. For example, an evaluation of the effectiveness of a particular rehabilitation team may show that services are less expensive, that the professionals on the team find their work more rewarding, and that agency administrators feel there is a better allocation of resources when a team approach is initiated. On the other hand, there may be no difference in patient progress or satisfaction with treatment. Whether such findings constitute "success" is a matter to be decided by those who request or initiate the evaluation. The use of appropriate evaluation procedures does not eliminate subjective judgment; it merely ensures that the data upon which such judgments are based are as accurate as possible.

2. **Which elements of the team approach lead to more effective outcomes?** If the team approach itself is the treatment which we are to evaluate, what variables of that treatment increase or decrease its effectiveness? Undoubtedly some kinds of teams are more effective than others. What factors make for significant differences in team functioning? What is it about that specific team that

is related to more successful treatment? Is it the use of case conferences, the recordkeeping system, the informal means of communication, the diversity of professional representation, or some other aspect of team functioning?

When a team approach is newly implemented, it is often found that some aspects work and others do not. Generally those elements that work are retained, and those that are less successful are dropped (either by design, or through gradual disuse). The task of evaluation is to determine more accurately which elements of the team approach are effective in a particular setting and which should be modified or eliminated. Unfortunately, it is often quite difficult to separate out the effect of various aspects, and the whole team approach may be evaluated negatively simply because of problems with *one* aspect.

3. **With which clients is the team approach most effective?** This question suggests a need to identify particular problems that are most amenable to a team approach. In Chapter 6 we noted that often the client's problems extend over a number of areas and must of necessity involve input from a variety of professions. In so far as the needs of the client define the team's task, we would expect that the team approach will prove more effective with certain populations.

4. **Under what conditions does the team operate most effectively?** We have already seen that the context in which the team operates may be an important factor in the team's effectiveness. What administrative support is needed if the team is to be successful? Are teams more successful in certain types of institutional settings or agencies than in others? Do teams function most effectively under particular administrative structures? These types of questions must be addressed in any evaluation project.

TYPES OF EVALUATION

The basic purpose of team evaluation is to improve decision making about the program, and to provide information for choosing between various courses of action. Should a particular team be continued in its present form, discontinued, or modified? This kind of decision is based on the results of evaluation research. As Weiss (1975) has described it:

> Evaluation research is a rational enterprise. It examines the effects of policies and programs on their targets (individuals, groups, institutions, communities) in terms of the goals they are meant to achieve. By objective and systematic methods, evaluation research assesses the extent to which goals are realized and looks at the factors associated with successful or unsuccessful outcomes. The assumption is that by providing the "facts," evaluation assists decision-makers to make wise choices among future courses of action. Careful and unbiased data on the consequences of the programs should improve decision-making (p. 13).

How to ensure the collection of such unbiased data is one of the major problems facing the evaluator. It should be noted that successful evaluation often requires the collection of a great deal of information. As Weinstein (1975) indicates, "while data about individuals served and the services they receive are the heart of the information system, other data must also be available" (p. 398). Among the "other data" Weinstein includes information about facility staff, organization of the facility, facility buildings, other resources used by the agency, finances and costs, and the geographic area served.

What procedures are available to help in the collection of data and the evaluation of a particular team operation? Although the methodological aspects of evaluation are not within the scope of this book, we will briefly examine two major approaches to evaluation and also look at some of the roles that seem to be appropriate in the evaluation of team effectiveness. More detailed information on evaluation procedures can be found in Anderson and Ball (1978), and Guttentag and Struening (1975).

Formative and Summative Evaluation

A useful distinction between two types of evaluation, formative and summative, has been made by Scriven (1967). Briefly, formative evaluation is used to help in the formation of a program by providing feedback on various components as the program develops, while summative evaluation assesses the overall effectiveness of a program after it is in operation. Formative evaluation research may include studies designed to pretest materials or measuring instruments, to collect data regarding characteristics of the target population, or to further define the goal of the program (Anderson, et al., 1975). Formative evaluation is usually an *internal* operation, or at least must be carried out in close cooperation with those designing and implementing the new program. Feedback is immediate and is used to modify the program *as it develops*. Results of a summative evaluation may be used to make decisions about modifying or eliminating a program *after the program has been developed and implemented.* Summative evaluation is often conducted by an outside evaluator who is independent of the program and can provide an objective assessment. Summative evaluation will often indicate intended and unintended positive and negative outcomes (Anderson, et al., 1975).

Both types of evaluation are appropriate forms of team research; which type should be used depends on the purpose of the evaluation and whether the team approach has already been implemented or is still in a planning or developmental stage. Formative evaluation may be thought of as a tracking device that provides feedback during the process. It operates like the radar controlled rocket which makes mid-course adjustments on the basis of a constant flow of information concerning its direction and speed. Summative evaluation on the other hand, operates like an artillery spotter who reports whether or not the shell hit the target and then advises corrections for the next shot.

The decision to use either formative or summative evaluation should be based upon the needs of the particular project or program to be evaluated. The advantage of formative evaluation consists of the possibility of intervention at an early stage, so that later stages of the operation will work better. Thus, the evaluation itself becomes part of the process. This aspect can also function as a disadvantage because it makes it almost impossible to say what would have occurred had the evaluation not been taking place. In the specific instance we are examining in this book, formative evaluation seems most suited to the evaluation of the team approach.

Summative evaluation looks at the end result. Since it is concerned only with end products, it has the advantage of not intervening in the process, thereby changing it and confounding the results. This is not to say that data cannot be collected during a project that is being evaluated — only that the evaluator does not intervene in the process.

Role of the Evaluator

In any project, program, or process that deals with the achievement of particular goals, there is a need to define the evaluator's role. This role may be filled by one or more persons. Those who accept this role must critically appraise the achievement of goals by means of a formative or summative evaluation. The evaluation must be designed and implemented in a manner consistent with the project and which will aid in the improvement of performance.

Techniques for data gathering and analysis should be consistent with good research practice. The role of evaluator demands not only technical expertise in the collection and analysis of data, but also interpersonal skill in conveying the results of evaluation. Evaluation is often looked upon with some trepidation by those being evaluated. Therefore, the evaluator must be skilled in handling what may be a very sensitive situation.

In some instances it may be best to employ an evaluator who is entirely removed from the program under study. The evaluator is presumably more objective if not related directly to the team and also may have a fresh point of view to bring to the evaluation. On the negative side, the evaluator may not have a complete understanding of the program or the time necessary to acquire the necessary background. Furthermore, he or she may not be available for follow-up on the recommendations stemming from the evaluation report.

The internal evaluator may not be so objective but is more likely to have the intimate knowledge of the program necessary to structuring an adequate evaluation. The internal evaluator is also assumed to have some commitment to the ongoing improvement of the team operation.

Accrediting agencies, government, and private funding agencies all make use of program reviews done by one's professional colleagues. One of the main problems with peer review is that peers do not always bring unbiased views to the review process and may be overly influenced by self-interest. Nevertheless, peer review is an important and much used method of evaluation.

RESEARCH

In addition to the need to evaluate the work of teams in particular institutions there is also a need for general research concerning teams. Such research would be facilitated by the development of a theory of teams as indicated in Chapter One. Certainly existing theory concerning groups and organizations may provide a framework for extending our knowledge of how teams function; however, as more and more data are amassed concerning teamwork, a more formal integrating construct is needed.

Briefly, a theory can be defined as a set of interrelated principles and definitions from which we derive specific hypotheses to test empirically. Such a theory has two basic functions:

1. to integrate existing knowledge
2. to suggest new relationships

and can be evaluated in terms of how well it fulfills those functions. The ultimate measure of a theory is not whether it is *true* (which we can never know), but whether it is *useful*. To the extent that a given theory organizes existing information and stimulates new research it may be regarded as a "good" theory.

As was pointed out earlier, there has been more rhetoric than research on the interdisciplinary team, and the research that has been conducted has been limited, spotty, and disorganized. The *team system* (Chapter One) provides one framework that suggests directions of future research. The three major aspects of the team system are the *components,* the *processes,* and the *outcomes* of the team. These aspects consist of:

Components	Processes	Outcomes
Client	Goals	Client
Professional	Activities	Professional
Organization	Task	Organizational
	Maintenance	Feedback

Each aspect presents us with a myriad of possible variables for investigation. With so many potential relationships to investigate, it may be difficult for the researcher to decide where to invest time and energy. From the team schema we have presented, three types of relationships are apparent. (This does not mean there are not other kinds of relationships or ways of looking at team research — we are simply suggesting one way in which one might proceed.) These relationships suggest several types of research problems.

Research Relating Components to Outcomes

This kind of research might focus, for example, on the impact of various organizational settings on the client. Do clients benefit more from the use of an interdisciplinary team than from alternative approaches? Is the treatment time shorter, does it cost less, is treatment more effective and is the client more satisfied as a result of the team approach? Similarly, what outcomes are there for professionals? Do they learn more and thus become better practitioners? Do they waste more or less time? Is job satisfaction greater or less? Does the organization benefit — is there better communication, fewer law suits?

Research Relating Components to Processes

Here we are looking at relationships between variables associated with the components and team processes. Research is needed on the way in which the personal and professional attributes of team members either enhance or detract from the effective operation of the team. Do various alternative organizational structures facilitate or impede team processes? How do interprofessional perceptions affect team interaction? Is it necessary for team members to "feel good" about the team for it to work well? Do certain types of leadership styles facilitate team goal setting?

Research Relating Processes to Outcomes

Here the processes would be related to variables associated with outcomes. One research area could involve an examination of the patterns of team interaction and cost effectiveness. Another might look at the way in which both task and maintenance goals are formulated in relation to both the activity of the team and the team's effectiveness in meeting the needs of the client, the professions, and the organization.

There has to date been little empirical observation of teamwork (Wagner, 1977). One would hope that additional research will be undertaken in the near future. The study of such questions is not without difficulty. As Nagi (1975) pointed out, there are a number of problems associated with studying teams, a prime one being the difficulty of defining and measuring quality of care. Associated with this are the problems of gaining access to data and the possible resistance to research by team members who may view such studies as a threat.

A different type of problem is that a good number of the people who have interest in the team as a research subject are strong *advocates* of the team approach. This may inhibit adequate research on the team as reflected by the large proportion of nonresearch based publications found by both Halstead and Wagner.

Another type of problem is that many would define as teams only those which operate exclusively on democratic, egalitarian principles. But many teams as defined in Chapter One do not operate on such principles and are in fact authoritarian in nature. Thus the "value set" of the researcher may lead him or her to collect data only on teams that operate in a certain way, and this too may inhibit research.

Finally, we suggest that the interdisciplinary team presents a unique opportunity for research, in that the research effort itself should probably be interdisciplinary, borrowing from methodologies used in a number of fields.

Chapter 9

Educating for Teamwork

If interdisciplinary teams are to function at an optimal level, professionals need to be trained or educated to function as part of a team. Of course, in order to function effectively as a team member, each professional must first be competent in his or her particular area of expertise. Training and practice in the field of specialization are necessary before an individual can make a major contribution to any team effort.

Once individuals are competent in their own professions, they must then develop competence in teamwork. The need for education in interdisciplinary team techniques has been recognized for some time. For instance, a report entitled "The participation of medical social workers in the teaching of medical students," published in 1939, stated that:

> The [medical] student will learn that resources can not be applied to needs in a categorical fashion, but that each patient's social problems must be regarded as individual and unique. He will further need to understand the possibilities and complexities of team work in caring for the patient whether between a number of skilled persons (such as physician, nurse, dietician and social worker) inside the hospital or between several agencies . . . . He will appreciate what he must know about community resources and about the methods of other professions which contribute to the patient's medical and social care. He will see how he must proceed in order to draw these others into such a plan or himself to cooperate with them if they turn to him for assistance on medical problems (Bartlett, 1939, p. 60).

This quotation demonstrates that the concept of educating for the team delivery of health care has been around for some time. However, early recognition of the concept has not always led to the development of such programs. For example, a survey of a sample of 175 professional schools including allied health, dentistry, nursing, medicine, and social work yielded the following results.

The overall response rate was 71 percent, with 124 schools responding. While 90 percent of the respondents replied affirmatively when questioned about the importance of having specific curricular provision for teaching the functions of the health care team, only 34 percent indicated that they now have such a course or unit of instruction in the curriculum. It should be noted that a few schools, particularly in the field of nursing, said that while they had no specific curricular provision for such instruction, it was "integrated" in present courses. In other words, while a large proportion of the respondents recognized the need for such educational offerings and 79 percent had considered such a course or unit, only 34 percent actually offered such a course. Indeed, in interviews with some schools that had such a course, it was found that the course was an elective and as such was often considered by the students to be peripheral to their real professional training.

In recent years professionals in many of the human service professions have shown increased interest in developing the means to improve the interdisciplinary team through education. A variety of specialities, including mental health, alcohol and drug abuse, rehabilitation and special education have espoused the concept of interdisciplinary education for teams. However, before exploring this concept further, let us examine briefly the need for understanding the competencies of other professions and some of the important factors in professional training.

UNDERSTANDING OTHER PROFESSIONS

A profession, as discussed in Chapter Two, is characterized by its unique body of knowledge. Indeed, if each member of the team did not possess unique information, theory, and skills, there would be little need for a team approach, except as a way of delegating work. The unique professional contribution of each team member is a major strength of the team approach. On the other hand, professionalization may at times be dysfunctional to the team effort in so far as it can lead to interprofessional conflict and misunderstanding.

Since most professionals are educated in a professionally segregated setting, there is usually little opportunity to understand the competencies of others. For adequate team functioning, team members should be familiar with other professions in order to best utilize coworkers' skills. As Devitt (1970) puts it:

> Better role definitions and better understanding of role functions by all members of the health team are necessary if health service is to become more efficient and more fruitful. The sloughing off of tasks by one health worker group to another further mandates better role function evaluation and better role definition. . . . Efforts in this direction are readily observable in each profession's journals, newsletters and convention proceedings (p. 6).

Devitt found that there was agreement among four health professions on 23 of 44 stated abilities related to professional competency, among them the ability to "analyze the strengths and limitation of his own professional role," to "distinguish major role functions of related professions," to "consult and coordinate with members of his and other professions as a means of achieving . . . health goals" (pp. 49-50), and to "recognize the importance of other health profession workers and the need for interlocking functions, responsibilities and esprit de corps" (p. 50). Devitt concludes that:

> A core curriculum might be a logical means for recruitment of individuals into a unified health professions program with the option of deferring specialty selection until students are more aware of role functions among various professions. . . . Another advantage of a core program is the greater opportunity it affords for interaction among beginning health professions students which should lead immeasurably to better interprofessional relationships following specialization (pp. 80-81).

While such an approach might seem sensible and promising in terms of economy, there is little hope that such an arrangement might be achieved. Patterns of curricula, professional structures, accreditation bodies, and institutional organizational patterns all seem to mitigate against this plan. However, such a core curriculum might be adopted on a more limited basis, through the identification of the shared competencies of the various professions and the use of common or cross-listed courses for each of the professional areas.

GOALS OF TEAM EDUCATION

While most professional education is aimed at developing an individual who can function autonomously and independently within an area of competence, team education seeks to develop one's ability to function interdependently with other professionals, using one's own skills and those of others in an optimum way. Education for teamwork is part of what has been termed interdisciplinary education. Szasz (1970) lists some objectives for the interdisciplinary team, including an increased awareness of need for a comprehensive approach; an understanding of the "attitudes, values and methods" of other professionals, as well as their skills; and an ability to use group dynamics in organizational relations.

Heilman (1977) reviewed the literature and conducted a number of interviews with experts in the field in order to identify the competencies needed by health care personnel to function as a health care team. This list of competencies was refined and reduced to 51 statements with relatively little overlap. These competencies were then rated by 20 experts as "of highest importance" to "of little importance or significance" for teamwork. Heilman concludes:

First priority among the 51 competencies was given to the need for a recognized leader for the team; the leader was not to be predetermined, but was to be selected by the group according to the task at hand. The ability of team members to handle conflicting personalities and divergent ideas was also given high importance. The health professional's perception of his own role, his security and self-confidence, were listed in the upper third [in importance]. Likewise, each one's understanding of the roles of other team members, of the differences in each one's perception of his role, and of the expertise possessed by each discipline on the team must be present if the team is to proceed harmoniously (p. 81).

Heilman discusses the need to develop training programs "to assure the acquisition and use of the teaming competencies, with systematic plans for developing the [highest rated] competencies," the importance of orienting faculty to a team approach to health care, and the "demand on administrators and organizations to plan for the initiation of the team approach" (Heilman, 1977, p. 82).

MODELS OF TEAM EDUCATION

Now that we have examined the need for interdisciplinary team education and some of its goals, let us look at some of the ways an education program dealing with teamwork might be provided. A variety of approaches can be envisioned, most of these variations of the same three models: preprofessional training, continuing education, and team development. *Preprofessional training* includes courses and programs in interdisciplinary teams designed for students as part of their professional training program. *Continuing education* programs include workshops and seminars in addition to formal coursework offered to professionals on an individual or group basis. *Team development* usually involves the use of consultants (either from within or from outside the agency) who work with an organization in order to initiate a new team or improve the operation of an existing team. Team development focuses on a specific team and helps the group analyze its functioning and make appropriate modifications in its operations.

Preprofessional Team Education

We have seen that a large proportion of deans of professional schools believe that educational preparation for teamwork is important, but most of the responding schools are not presently offering such coursework. Many advocates of team education believe the appropriate time for such training is during the period of basic professional preparation. This is a traditional approach that has often been used when innovations in professional practice suggest that an important content area or particular skill that is needed by the professional in the field is not being provided in the curriculum.

There are three elements of interdisciplinary team education at the preprofessional level:

1. cognitive (primarily didactic) information — including organizational theory, small group dynamics, and the sociology of the professions

2. affective (and experiential) learning — by participating in a team, the students learn through experience how a team operates, how roles are established, how leadership emerges, etc.

3. clinical training — By participating as part of a team in assessment, treatment, and similar activities with the client, the student not only learns necessary clinical skills but also learns how to use those skills in conjunction with other professionals. These skills may vary not only with profession (e.g., nursing, counseling, special education), but also with the type of situation in which the student is placed (a neighborhood clinic, a special classroom, a hospital, etc.).

Team education programs at the preprofessional level may concentrate on one, two, or all three of these aspects. For example, Infante, Speranza, and Gillespie (1976) report the development of a didactic interdisciplinary course with an experiential component in which the students work on a course project in small groups. Harris, Saunders, and Zasorin-Connors (1978) report an effort at the Medical College of Virginia where students participated in both didactic and experiential work during an eight-week elective course. In that course the experiential portion consisted of assessing the health care needs of a selected group of families and referring them to appropriate community agencies. Other courses have developed programs in which students are given interdisciplinary team assignments in various kinds of clinical settings and work collaboratively to provide services to clients. These clinical experiences generally cover certain theoretical material as well as give some attention to team dynamics within the group. In these types of programs, students *learn about* teams (cognitive), *work in* teams (affective), and *treat clients* (clinical). This seems to be a total approach to team education.

The authors have conducted a course in The Division of Interdisciplinary Programs of the School of the Health Related Professions, University of Pittsburgh. The course considers the variables that influence the team, such as professional roles; organizational settings; group dynamics; communication; legal, social, and financial factors. Students are expected to:

- demonstrate the ability to identify competencies and use other professionals in an interdisciplinary team

- describe the impact of various organizational settings on team functioning

- analyze and evaluate the influence of team dynamics and of various subcultural factors (such as professional roles and status) on the functions of an interdisciplinary team

- evaluate various models for educating team members in the function of teams and team development

- analyze and evaluate models of team decision making

- demonstrate the ability to communicate effectively with other team members (including patients, professionals, and paraprofessionals), and function in appropriate roles within the team

The course includes didactic work (principally lecture/discussion of pertinent research) and an experiential component in which each student is assigned to a team within the class. The student teams are then required to develop unified reports on an operational team located in a facility within the region. This seems to be an economical means of having the students experience some of the opportunities and frustrations of teamwork. The teams are asked to develop reports on the basis of direct observations of the team they have chosen, along with interviews of various team members. Teams that have been studied have ranged from a neurosurgical team to an emergency medical rescue unit. Students in the course have come from 15 different professions.

Evaluation of the course has indicated that the participants feel the project is rewarding but frustrating in that they are forced to work together to achieve the goals of the course (50 percent of the grade is based on the project). The instructors unobtrusively but systematically observe the teams and intervene only when a high-conflict situation arises. The final examination covers the didactic work and includes an item asking the participants to analyze the development of their team. Answers to this item have indicated that almost all of the participants were able to use the principles taught in the course to better perceive the dynamics of their particular team.

Although there have been a number of preprofessional courses and programs in interdisciplinary education throughout the country, special mention should be made of the Institute for Health Team Development at Montifiore Hospital and Medical Center in New York City. The Institute "is involved in working out a curriculum for the training of health science students from various disciplines whose goal is to provide family-centered primary care as members of a health team" (Bufford and Kindig, 1974, p. 149). Although focusing on primary care, many of the findings of the Institute projects have implications for interdisciplinary teams in other settings. The Institute initially conducted training in interdisciplinary education for faculty teams at a number of universities throughout the country (including the University of Washington, the University of North Carolina, and the University of Kentucky) and then assisted those schools in establishing interdisciplinary courses for students in the health professions. The university programs involve a number of professional schools such as medicine, dentistry, nursing, social work, allied health, and pharmacy, and provide both didactic and experiential components. Usually a clinical experience is also included.

There are a number of barriers that have to be overcome before effective preprofessional interdisciplinary education programs can be designed. The *institutional barriers* may be administrative, academic, logistic (time, cost), and attitudinal. *Individual barriers* include those associated with the acculturation of the individual to the profession, one professional's perception of another, and the trainee's background (socioeconomic status, level of training, and goals).

There may be a number of administrative problems in negotiating and managing an interdisciplinary program involving several professional schools. Not only may the schools have different ideas of what should be taught, they may even teach at different times. Often professional schools are on schedules of varying lengths, so it is difficult to accommodate students from several different schools.

The questions of *what* to teach and *how* to teach it are equally important. The faculty must decide whether the team education component will focus on cognitive aspects (through didactic material), affective aspects (with an experiential component), or both. Will the program take place in an academic or clinical setting? Faculty may be divided on how the program should be implemented, and the schools involved may have conflicting values on this issue. Although a program may ideally provide all components simultaneously, it may be difficult for the students to benefit from this approach. It may be that learning the theoretical basis for teamwork, in addition to learning how to interact with clients and with other professional team members is so overwhelming that the student actually retains very little. Furthermore, most students are engaged in other coursework at the same time and may feel overloaded and not able to commit sufficient energy to the program.

Team education is often introduced as part of an existing course or as a new course. If the coursework is felt to be sufficiently significant, the new area becomes part of the required "core" of professional training in that discipline. This means either expanding the requirements of the professional program or eliminating another area that was previously required. Since programs cannot continually add requirements, eventually the addition of new areas means the elimination of old requirements.

The new area may also be competing with other innovative areas in the field as well as with existing curricular requirements. Thus attempts to modify the curricula of professional schools often leads to a serious examination of priorities within the program. "We just can't teach them everything they need to know" is a frequent lament heard in curriculum committees.

What *is* taught may at times be based primarily on political considerations within the school or be included because of pressures exerted by professional organizations or clinicians in the field. Particularly in periods of rapid change, there is likely to be some confusion regarding which innovations are "fads" and which are likely to become a permanent part of the repertoire of professional behaviors. For example, when behavior modification was first introduced into professional practice, many psychologists, counselors, and teachers saw it as just another fad. At the present time, however, some knowledge of behavior modification is generally required in professional preparation programs. More and more professional schools seem to be taking the position that the interdisciplinary team approach is a genuine innovation and not just another professional fad.

The numbers of students and the lack of a place to put them are two common logistical problems which must be overcome in instituting interdisciplinary education. One such problem is pointed to by Rocereto (1977) in evaluating what appeared to be a successful pilot project with a student team in a neighborhood health center.

> It did not appear feasible to replicate the . . . experience on a large scale
> . . . one reason was . . . the project was costly in resources. Approximately 16 primary care sites would be needed year round to provide . . .
> clinical experience for all health professions students. In addition to shortage of sites, difficulties would be encountered in scheduling students from different schools for the same time period.

Costs were also mentioned as one of the reasons for not expanding the project. There would be a need for faculty participators at the site as well as additional program directors.

The faculty involved in planning and implementing an interdisciplinary team program may experience many of the same problems in working together as do the members of a direct service team. They too, must work together as a team, negotiate, and learn to understand each other's roles and capabilities. At the same time, the primary responsibilities of these faculty rest in their own professional school. Thus, despite a striking commitment often found in those involved in team education, the realities of their position and limited time and energy may severely restrict what can actually be done.

Finally, a serious problem we have noted with preprofessional team training is that new professionals are still unsure of their own developing professional skills and their roles vis-à-vis other professionals. While a number of authors have noted the problems for interdisciplinary teamwork created by early socialization in the profession during preprofessional training (Bufford and Kindig, 1974; Frank, 1961; Lewis and Resnick, 1966), the other side of this coin is that lack of confidence in one's own professional skills may make it more difficult to interact with other professionals early in the training experience. We have found that students in our classes who are not yet sure "who they are" professionally sometimes have difficulty interacting with other more advanced students in other professions. Erikson contends in his theory of human development (1963) that true intimacy comes only after the individual has developed a secure sense of identity and can "let go" of that identity sufficiently to merge with another. While interdisciplinary team relationships are considerably less intense than the kinds of relationships Erikson had in mind, it may well be that students are not ready to profit fully from an interdisciplinary team experience until they have developed sufficient clinical or professional skills to have some degree of confidence in their identities and abilities. Only then can they truly represent their profession to other members of the team so that all can learn from each other.

At the present time, most team educators seem to support the idea of early interdisciplinary training. In a discussion of why professionals find it difficult to work together, Bufford and Kindig (1974) develop a rationale for introducing team education early in professional training.

> One of the most important [reasons] is that the training of doctors, nurses, social workers, family health workers, etc. is generally confined to contacts with members of the same professional group. These people have little opportunity to get to know professionals from other disciplines until "professional roles" have been pretty much internalized. Furthermore, these professionals have not been taught *how* to work collaboratively.
>
> The result is that students of various disciplines enter into patient care experiences with preset expectations of each other's roles and capabilities. Such expectations tend to lock into a continued cycle of traditional interactions between professional and professional, and professional and patient. This not only weakens the educational potential but also, ultimately, the service capabilities of health professionals — at the expense, of course, of the patient (pp. 150-151).

The need for interdisciplinary experiences early in professional training was also identified by Lewis and Resnick (1966) on the basis of the results of an interdisciplinary clinical elective for medical and nursing students. They found that, contrary to expectations, the objectives of the two groups did not become more similar as a result of the interdisciplinary experience, and the authors attributed this finding to professional socialization early in the student's training.

Kindig (1975) recommends an interdisciplinary seminar be included early in the professional education of health science students. Hudson and Giacalone (1975), in discussing collaborative courses, also suggest "ideally such programs should be introduced as early as possible into the curriculum for all types of students . . . " (p. 215) with provisions for reintroducing some materials after students have developed clinical skills and have a better perspective of their own roles in the team. However, the authors caution that "the concept of multiprofessional student collaborative education has not been universally accepted and frank skepticism is expressed by some" (215).

With regard to collaborative clinical experiences, Hudson and Giacalone conclude, "it is suggested that students from the various health professions at the point in their education where they would normally be scheduled for clinical experience should be introduced, whenever possible, into clinical settings which fully incorporate team processes" (p. 216).

Educational institutions must decide what priority will be placed on interdisciplinary teamwork in the professional curriculum. Once the decision is made, the institutional and individual barriers to the development of adequate approaches may be addressed. Thus far although a number of professionals support the concept, there have been significantly few who have been able to initiate and maintain programs.

Continuing Education

Continuing education programs are one means of upgrading professional skills and imparting knowledge of current research and innovative techniques to practicing professionals in a wide variety of fields. It reaches those who did not receive training in teamwork during their preprofessional education and gives further training to those who did. A major advantage of continuing education programs is that the practicing professional who sees the need for additional skills in a particular area is highly motivated to learn.

While many educators fear that the established professional may lack sufficient role flexibility for effective teamwork, it is also possible that the professional's knowledge of and confidence in his or her own role (as well as the roles of other professionals) may prove to be an advantage in a team education program.

It seems apparent, however, that if professionals are to be adequately educated for effective team interaction, both preprofessional and continuing educational programs are needed. Although there have been several different kinds of workshops and seminars offered, one of the most ambitious has been that of the Center for Interdisciplinary Education in Allied Health at the University of Kentucky. In addition to sponsoring a number of preprofessional and continuing education projects, the Center has been involved in the development of materials for the training of team members.

The goals of the Center are stated in its progress report:

> The Center exists as a resource unit to health science educational programs which desire to begin or improve their efforts in teaching an interdisciplinary (team) approach to the delivery of health care. The resources of the Center will be directed towards research in teaching interdisciplinary (team) concepts; development and preparation of educational materials and evaluation methodologies, providing a focal point for information on interdisciplinary (team) educational activities; and providing laboratory experiences for teachers and students in an active interdisciplinary setting.
>
> The philosophy and activities of the Center for Interdisciplinary Education in Allied Health lead to its two goals:
>
> 1. To be a catalytic agent for the development and implementation of interdisciplinary activities in health science programs, particularly Allied Health.
> 2. To be a research and development center for teaching/learning methodology and evaluation in interdisciplinary education in the health sciences.
>
> Recognizing that Allied Health personnel do not work in isolation from other disciplines, it is expected that the Center will be available to work with educational units of other health science disciplines outside those popularly classified as Allied Health (Connelly, 1978).

Another example, albeit representative of a more limited approach, are the one-day workshops designed by the authors to address the team-related problems of the participants. Specifically, workshop goals invite the participants to:

1. examine the rationale, concepts, and basic principles of the interdisciplinary team
2. explore barriers to satisfactory team performance
3. develop methods for improving team effectiveness.

In addition to lecture/discussion of the team system, the participants are asked to provide a set of critical incidents they have observed that illustrate ineffective team performance. These incidents are then discussed and categorized. For example, at one workshop the critical incidents yielded the following distribution:

Common Barriers to Team Effectiveness

Organizational structure	23.4%
Goal conflict	14.8%
Interpersonal and interprofessional conflict	26.2%
Communication	35.5%

Further discussion then points up the need for role negotiation and better attention to communication patterns. The impingement of organizational structure on team operations and some approaches to conflict management are also discussed.

Evaluation of the workshops indicated that the participants thought the workshops were for the most part useful in helping them understand their teams and making them aware of the ways to improve team performance.

The continuing education approach holds a great deal of promise in that it can reach those practitioners who are most concerned with improving the effectiveness of team operation. It may also be less expensive than alternative approaches.

One problem is the question of impact or effectiveness in the actual improvement of team performance. Most continuing education programs tend to be of short duration — one to three days. They bring together persons from a number of agencies or professions, deal with a specific topic, and send the participants back to work. The assumption, of course, is that the individual will be able to apply what has been learned to the work situation. Unfortunately, there is little follow-up on this point.

Team Development

According to Rubin and Beckhard (1972):

> If a health team is first to survive and second to grow, it must develop an attitude and a capability for building and renewing itself as a team. It can do this first by becoming aware of how its internal group processes influence its ability to function and second by learning how to manage these processes or maintenance needs in a more productive manner (p. 328).

As they see it, team development focuses on the group processes of the team, helping members look at the goals, norms, tasks, decision making, etc., of the team, with periodic "check-ups" to ensure that the team is functioning effectively. Although some of the training (in leadership skills, for example) can be conducted during individual professional preparation, "some training needs to be done with the team as a unit" (p. 333). Furthermore, since older teams may be less flexible, Rubin and Beckhard suggest that perhaps team development should take place as early as possible after the formation of a team. As they point out:

Early team development efforts would have several distinct advantages: (a) the period of initial socialization has a significant effect on the team's future development — early experiences set a very strong tone that influences future events; (b) a group can more easily create the kind of culture, norms and procedures it deems useful if it is starting fresh rather than having to "undo" a long history of past experiences; (c) perhaps most important would be the early recognition that the team really has two equally important tasks — to deliver health care and to continuously work to develop and maintain itself as a well-functioning team to improve its services (p. 333).

Another effort in team development has been the work of Rubin, Plovnick, and Fry (1975) entitled, *Improving the Coordination of Care: A Program for Health Team Development.* This program is based on a number of pilot projects with teams at the Martin Luther King, Jr. Health Center, and is described by its authors as:

A program of task-oriented activities aimed at helping any group of health workers and/or administrators responsible for the delivery of health care to get its job done in the most effective way possible. This program focuses on specifically defining the job that needs to get done and procedures for doing it. The program requires seven three-hour periods of the work-group's time and requires no outside consultant (p. 1).

There is much to be said about the advantages and disadvantages of the team development approach. Among the principle advantages is that the work can be directed to the specific problems of a team, giving little or no emphasis to areas of team operation that are working smoothly. Secondly, the persons who participate in team development are able to increase their awareness of how their own team and teams in general function.

One disadvantage is that this approach may be costly in time and money without yielding much apparent improvement in the way team tasks are addressed and completed. If outside consultants are asked to aid in team development it is imperative that sufficient time be taken to evaluate what the team actually needs and address those needs in a non-destructive manner. For instance, one workshop participant told the story of a team that was functioning fairly well until a consultant was called in to improve their operation. What happened was "he came in and in just one day took us apart. We never did get together again in the two years I was at the agency." The talented consultant should at very least do no harm, but the inept consultant may create or exacerbate problems that will remain long after she or he is gone.

A more extensive review of team development methods is found in Chapter Ten.

Finally, one of the most striking aspects of professional education is that we are presently training people for roles they will continue to fill 20 or 30 years from now. Not only must we make educated guesses about the skills and competencies that will be needed by professionals in the future, we must also develop in our students a flexibility that will allow them to shift roles and responsibilities as conditions in their fields change.

Since it seems that the interdisciplinary team will continue to be an important aspect of health care delivery in the coming years, it is likely that preprofessional preparation for teamwork will become more common and that there will also be a growing need for expanded programs of continuing education and team development.

Chapter 10

Improving Team Performance

Throughout this book we have been concerned with those factors that affect the performance of an interdisciplinary team and the services it provides to clients in health care and other human service settings. Two major functions of the team, task-related activities and team maintenance activities, have been identified and explored. These two functions are obviously related, since time and energy devoted to one is then not available for the other. To the extent that the team must spend time and energy in organizing itself to complete the task and in dealing with interpersonal relationships, there will be a loss in efficiency, referred to as *process loss* (Steiner, 1972). According to Steiner, this loss is the difference between the *potential* productivity of the group (given the demands of the task and the resources of the group) and its *actual* productivity. Thus in some ways interaction may hinder the performance of the task.

On the other hand, according to Hackman and Morris (1975), there are also some potential *process gains* as a result of group interaction. Although these gains sometimes go unrecognized, they make it possible for the group to achieve a more effective outcome than might have been anticipated from knowledge about individual members. For example, group interaction may increase the amount of effort members are willing to expend, increase the total pool of knowledge available, and help the group develop strategies for carrying out the task. Thus by working cooperatively, group members may arrive at solutions that are better than the sum of the members' independent efforts. This of course, is the reason for using the team approach.

The extent of both process loss and process gains (i.e., the actual effectiveness of the group) will be determined by a number of factors. As Steiner (1972) indicates, the productivity of the group depends on the demands of the task, the resources available to the group, and the process of the group. We have discussed how increasing the size and the heterogeneity of a team may increase the resources available. But at the same time, by increasing the complexity of the interpersonal

167

interactions, process loss may also be increased. In previous chapters we have also examined some of the processes in which teams engage and how these may affect outcomes of the team. In this chapter we will review several aspects of the team system that may create barriers to team performance, and suggest methods that may be used to reduce them.

PROFESSIONS

Professionalization can present a number of barriers to the development of the team. The professional has been educated to act as an autonomous individual, and the team as a system takes from the professional some degree of autonomy. This can be a barrier to team effectiveness. Linked to *autonomy* is the notion of *specialization*, which in effect supports the impetus to act alone without reference to others who may be treating the patient.

In order to deal with the questions of professional autonomy and specialization it is necessary to first discover how both factors are perceived by team members. The boundaries of professional responsibility are not clearcut, and perhaps some team time should be spent on the question: Where does my ability to autonomously decide what treatment will be accorded to a patient start and end?

For example, one administrator of a nursing home indicated that he had a physician and a pharmacist as part of his team and that the physician continually overruled and/or ignored the pharmacist's suggestions concerning appropriate medications. Ignoring for the moment the question of who is right or wrong, there certainly is a need for these two professionals to address their differences.

Often this type of question can be confronted at a team meeting designed to deal with the question of professional responsibilities and prerogatives. Such an agenda may do much to clear the air concerning who does what and who decides who does what. However, care must be taken in structuring such meetings so that they do not become just another battleground for interprofessional conflict. At times it is helpful to develop subgroups within the team to tackle the question of how two or more professions can work together in everyone's best interests. This process may be mediated by a third person who understands the professions involved and has no personal axe to grind. Such mini-consultations can focus on various groupings of individuals and professionals without involving all the team at once. Often such an approach seems less threatening to those involved, if the need for such meetings is first discussed in a general way with the total team.

Topics to be discussed include but are not limited to professional autonomy, specialization, division of labor, delegation of authority and responsibility, the knowledge base of the various professions, and professional stereotypes. If such a discussion is treated as a *routine exercise* in improving team function, with the assumption that no one of the professions adequately understands the skills and competencies of another, much will be done to dispel the common concern among professionals that they "really should know what X profession can contribute but would be embarrassed to ask," or that they "really do know the abilities and skills of X profession" but in point of fact do not.

One useful exercise concerning professional roles and stereotypes can be developed using the Interprofessional Perception Scale (IPS). Since the instrument is essentially based on "how I see you, how I think you see yourself, and how I think that you think I see you," it can be an excellent takeoff point for discussing a number of areas of interprofessional interaction. Subjects such as ethics, competence status, autonomy, and interprofessional understanding are addressed. Of course, care should be taken to explain the purpose of using the IPS and explain also the differences in perception that are uncovered. Sometimes it is best to have individuals complete the IPS anonymously and tabulate the results in the same way, using group data to stimulate discussion. At other times it is best to use data from more general populations, thus depersonalizing the responses and thereby reducing to some extent the threat to those present. (As additional IPS data becomes available, it will be made available to appropriate users.)

Another aspect of professionalization that sometimes creates a barrier to effective team operation is the question of *ethical standards.* As was pointed out in Chapter Three, the various human services professions differ considerably in the content of their professional codes of ethics. To a large extent the differences may be the result of professional territoriality. Such differences make it difficult to generalize from one code to another. Some codes of ethics ignore the team as an approach to patient care. This is especially true on the subject of sharing information concerning clients; if observed to the letter, some professional codes of ethics in effect preclude some professionals from participating in teams. Some codes also fail to provide clearcut standards governing the activities of nonprofessionals on the team.

It would seem appropriate that the various professional organizations that promulgate codes of ethics might convene to discuss the effects of those codes on interdisciplinary approaches to health care. Until that happens, however, it will be necessary for individual team members to interpret their codes to other team members so that there will be mutual understanding of the constraints such standards impose. Since some professions have more highly developed codes of ethics than others, it would seem appropriate that these groups use their knowledge to help others refine and develop their own codes.

A related problem is that of differential *legal responsibility* for the client. Briefly, it is necessary for the various professionals on a team to ascertain their individual and joint legal responsibilities. It should be remembered that although the team approach seems to diffuse responsibility, it does not necessarily abrogate individual responsibility. Such clarification may do much to improve relationships between team members when decisions must be made and responsibility for performance fixed.

A highly sensitive area of interprofessional relationships is *status*. An individual's status is often determined to a large extent by her or his profession. Status influences communications, decision making, and the overall operation of the team. It is generally best to openly recognize professional hierarchies and discuss their possible impact on team functioning; this does much to mitigate against their negative influences over time.

One negative influence is often found in the area of communication: those more junior on the status scale tend to defer to others of higher status even when they have better and more accurate information concerning the problem at hand. One way to alleviate this problem is to establish clear protocols of operation that reward participation in information giving and decision making.

In summary, to enhance its operations the team should attend to several areas related to professionalization:

- Autonomy
- Specialization
- Division of tasks
- Ethics
- Delegation of authority
- Knowledge base and overlaps
- Roles and stereotypes
- Legal responsibilities
- Status

Areas that present problems should be addressed by a number of different techniques, such as:

- Information sharing in groups and between individuals
- Mediated small group information sessions
- General information sessions

Each of these techniques should be used in a planned, orderly fashion that precludes the notion that "something is wrong." Indeed, there should be an open indication that to improve the performance of any team it is necessary to address a number of operational factors on a regular basis. If this attitude is accepted by team members, team development becomes a normal and effective *process* rather than a crisis, confrontation *event*.

THE CLIENT

We have emphasized throughout this book that the team is essentially client centered; that is, that the client is the primary focus of the team's attention. This does not rule out the possibility that at times the client may actually raise barriers that interfere with the effective functioning of the team. In fact it is *because* clients play such a central role in the team system that they can create such major difficulties.

Client-Related Barriers

In Chapter Four we looked at a few studies describing the expectations professionals hold for "good" patients. The work of Lorber (1975), for example, indicated that hospital staff saw "problem patients" as those who demand a great deal of attention. When patients are seriously ill they are not held responsible for their demands, but patients who demand attention solely through complaints and uncooperative behavior may actually receive less adequate services because of the staff's attitudes.

Not only the "problem patient," but other stereotyped patient types, may also hinder the team's efforts, directly or indirectly. Let us look briefly at some of the ways these patient-helper interactions may reduce the team effectiveness. Four patterns can be identified, along with some techniques for coping with them.

The Problem Patient

A prototype of the problem patient is Mr. Jones, mentioned in Team Conference A in Chapter Six. That this patient is considered a problem by the team is often recognizable by the members' reaction when the client's name is brought up in the team meeting. Certainly, some team discussion of the problems raised by such patients may serve to diffuse some of the negative feelings staff members develop in working with them. Sometimes information contributed by other team members can in part explain some of the client's deviant behavior and may help change the team's attitudes toward the client. It is particularly important that the team leader keep discussion of the problem patient within reasonable bounds so that the team's resentment and frustration do not become exacerbated by the team meeting rather than alleviated through the discussion. The team leader can help the group maintain some degree of objectivity toward the client, and most important, *avoid decisions about the patient that are essentially punitive rather than treatment-focused*.

The Manipulative Client

The client who is accused of being manipulative is one who is adept at playing off one team member against another, in the same way that children sometimes learn to pit mother against father. "Dr. Smith said I could leave the hospital this afternoon" may be a straightforward statement of a fact, or it may be a subtly distorted version of what Dr. Smith actually said (or didn't say). Like the problem patient, the manipulative client may evoke a host of negative emotions from various members of the team. However, the team approach intrinsically offers certain advantages in working with patients who seek to play on the inconsistencies of the system. If the team has agreed on a course of action and team members jointly support the plan, there should be fewer contradictions and inconsistencies for such a client to seize on. More important, the team meetings can help staff members better understand the needs of certain clients to maintain a sense of control when placed in what may be helpless and dependent positions. The team may be able to identify other legitimate ways the patient can exert power in the system without resorting to game playing.

Sometimes staffers' perceptions of the patient are so different that misunderstanding can easily develop. Some team members may be overly protective of the client, while other members feel that such behavior is "naive and unprofessional." These issues may need to be addressed directly by the team leader before the dissatisfaction can spread. In any case, the client should not become a divisive factor that disrupts the cohesiveness of the team.

The Yea-Sayer

The "yea saying" client is one who is unusually compliant in responding to the team's efforts. While this may sound like the behavior of a "good" client, in fact the client's excessively compliant and passive behavior may at times cause problems for the team. Just as a shy and withdrawn child may be overlooked in a classroom of aggressive fifth graders, so the client who always accepts whatever the professionals say may not be receiving adequate attention from the team. Team meetings may focus on clients who are management problems of one sort or another, and the yea-sayer simply does not come up. A schedule for reviewing clients can ensure that every client receives some attention at the team conference.

Another problem with yea-saying clients is that it may be difficult to determine just what the clients themselves want. Their tendency to agree with every suggestion made by the staff can lead to considerable confusion and even conflict around goal setting and long term planning. As with the manipulative client, it is particularly important that the team agree on a consistent course of action. Otherwise, it might be discovered that the client has agreed to two or more different, perhaps even inconsistent, plans.

The Unmotivated Client

In truth there is no such thing as an unmotivated client, since any client who is alive — eating, breathing, sleeping — is obviously motivated. The label generally refers to a client who is not motivated to the degree expected or in the direction expected by the team. Such clients tend to be the source of considerable frustration and may even elicit widespread hostility among team members. The ultimate punishment for the unmotivated client is discharge from the program or agency. "We want to make room for another client who will get more out of being here," is the comment frequently heard. In many circumstances this is a reasonable alternative for the team to consider.

Sometimes however, spending some time on the problem in a team conference will lead to a better understanding of the client's dynamics and resulting behavior. Perhaps the client is acting out of anxiety and fear of failure, and by not really trying the failure is averted. In other cases, lack of incentives rather than lack of motivation may be the crucial factor. Working together, the team may be able to reduce the client's anxiety, provide appropriate rewards, or modify the environment in some way so that the client can cope more effectively with the demands of the agency and the expectations of the team.

When teams use labels such as "manipulative" or "unmotivated" in referring to clients, team members sometimes get the impression that the client's behavior has somehow been "explained." It is important to recognize that such labels add nothing to an understanding of the client's problems; the labels should not become an excuse for inaction. "Since she isn't motivated, we really can't do anything for her," is a common statement. The team can serve to explain to its members the danger of using vague generalizations as a basis for decision making and can provide a broader information base on which decisions can be made.

The Client as Team Member

One way to obviate many of the client-related barriers described above is to include the client as a team member. As active participants in the discussions concerning their problems, clients can have major input in the decision process. Compliant patients can be asked to choose between alternatives, the complaints of the problem patient can be aired, and the game playing of the manipulative client can be dealt with directly. On the other hand, some professionals on the team feel uncomfortable when patients are present at the team meeting and may hesitate to raise certain issues unless they have been discussed beforehand with other professionals on the team.

It is important to clarify the client's role on the team in order to avoid misunderstandings that may otherwise arise. Whether clients are always included in team meetings concerning their problems, included only when circumstances demand their presence, or never included, is a policy decision that deserves discussion. The policy most appropriate for a particular team depends on a number of factors including the type of population served, the makeup of the team, and the policies of the organization. Similarly, teams that deal frequently with parents or other family members also need to examine the role of the family as it interacts with the team.

In summary then, the team may wish to address these questions:

- How is the deviant client typically dealt with by the team?
- What role is the client expected to play on the team — passive recipient or active participant?
- Are parents or other family members expected to participate in team decision making? If so, how?

ORGANIZATIONS

Organizations differ in detail but are similar in general characteristics. As has been pointed out, the pervasive organizational pattern in the Western world is bureaucratic. Given this type of structure, the impact of the organization upon team functions begins to take on more meaning and greater clarity. The interface between the organization and the team makes it necessary to attend to those aspects of the interaction that may be dysfunctional. Goals and objectives, power and authority, process and procedures, and rewards and sanctions are among those aspects that have influence upon team operations. As discussed in Chapter Five, the individual organizational setting has much to do with the way the team is organized and functions.

The major question to be faced by any organization that espouses team principles for the delivery of human services is *commitment*. Is the organization willing to alter itself in such a way as to nurture and enhance the team function? If not, then the parent organization, if it is typically bureaucratic, will be at constant odds with the team or teams within it. This is because the organization is built up along the same divisions of labor as the professions. It tends to emphasize and reinforce the divisions between disciplines and tends to restrict communication along hierarchical lines. Rewards and sanctions tend to be delivered through the same channels and for the same reasons. Teams, on the other hand, tend to be structured so as to emphasize the sharing of knowledge and communication across disciplines. Suffice it to say that any organization that seriously comtemplates the development of effective teams must answer the following questions:

- Are the goals and objectives of the organization as a whole adequately communicated to the team structure? Are they understood?
- Are the goals and objectives of the team and the organization shared?

If the team does not share the goals of the parent organization, some accommodation must be reached. Either the goals are not appropriate, or the team has not been integrated into the organizational structure.

- How is team membership defined?
- Are appropriate roles assigned by the organization?
- Is there ambiguity as to role? If so, how is this resolved within the organizational structure?

One of the main purposes of organization is to control and direct human behavior. The assignment of tasks and roles and the definition of what constitutes membership are important activities of any organization. The relationship between role definition and activity in a team system is crucial to the functions of the team.

- How is the authority structure of the organization reflected in the team? (Who decides? Who decides who decides)?

It is imperative for adequate team functioning that the authority structure reinforce the activities of the team. Crucial here is the position of the team leader in relation to the organization as a whole. What kinds of decisions can a team leader make? How are they enforced? May they be overruled? Does the team fit with the formal authority structure or does the authority of the team evolve from other sources (such as from the individual personal or professional attributes of its members)? For example, if a particular team member is considered to be "the" expert in a particular field, it is likely that a team decision in that area would not be overlooked or overruled by persons who hold normative authority within the organization.

- How is the team integrated into the pattern of communication within the organization?
- Are the systems of record keeping, storage, and retrieval of information consonant with team organization?
- Are there organizational barriers to effective communication from and to teams?

When teams are made up of a number of professionals, each from a separate unit of an organization, it may be that organization-team communication is assumed to occur because of the dual membership. This is not necessarily true. Therefore, an analysis of communication patterns is an important and useful step in improving team and organizational performance.

- How do processes, rules, and procedures fit with team operation?

Each organization has some fundamental processes by which it works to fulfill its goals. Such processes may not facilitate team functioning since they originated when teams did not exist. A careful look at the way organization processes, rules, and procedures enhance or deter team functioning is in order.

- How do the reward/sanction systems relate to the team?
- What are the norms and values of the organization in relation to the team?

Perhaps no other area of organizational function is so important to team success as the system of rewards and sanctions imposed by the organization. If teamwork and team effort are not rewarded in some way, the team system will not function. The expected normative behavior of the individual in the organization as well as the informal value system also influence the way in which the team functions. These aspects should be critically appraised when attempting team improvement.

- Does the arrangement of space (e.g., offices, conference rooms) enhance or detract from team efficiency?

While it is often overlooked, the spatial arrangement of an organization can do much to either enhance or detract from the effective team operation. Territoriality and space can have a significant bearing on human interaction: proximity generally enhances communication.

- What evaluation procedures are used? How do they relate to the team?

In any organization, evaluation of activities closely reflects what is perceived as being valued and rewarded within the institution. The evaluation procedures must take into account the team system, or the system will of consequence suffer.

While this list of questions is by no means exhaustive, it does provide a starting place for examining how the team interacts with the organization. A careful examination, based on these parameters, may be helpful in uncovering areas where work must be done.

GOAL DEFINITION AND GOAL CONFLICTS

In Chapter Six we indicated the need to clearly define team goals and identify goal conflicts that may potentially disrupt the team. Team members need to ask:

- Are team goals and objectives adequately defined?
- Is there a consensus among team members regarding priorities for the team?

These questions are relevant not only for new teams in their early stages of development, but also for teams that have been in existence for some time.

The newly formed team may experience the greatest difficulty with defining goals, since initial goal statements are often rather vague and fuzzy. A goal definition exercise of some kind can help sort out the perceptions of various team members regarding goals and indicate the directions in which the team sees itself moving.

The team that is already functioning may experience some difficulty in the area of goal conflict. Team members may unknowingly hold quite different notions of some of the team goals, and this may lead to repeated disagreements regarding appropriate courses of action to be taken by the team. Again, a goal definition exercise can help identify hidden conflicts in team goals and provide a basis for negotiating and redefining those goals.

Goal Definition Exercise

The following exercise is one the authors have found useful with newly formed and with existing teams. By comparing the goal perceptions of various team members, areas of consensus and disagreement can be identified and discussed, and priorities can be determined. The exercise has two phases and involves the following steps:

Phase One

1. Each team member is asked to briefly write out *three major goals of the team*. Each goal statement is written on a separate 3 x 5 card. Participants do not sign their names to the goal cards.

2. The goal cards are collected by the team leader or a designated person (who need not be a team member), shuffled to ensure a random order, and numbered. Then *each card is read to the group*.

3. In this first "run-through" of the goal cards, the participants are asked to sort each statement into one of four categories: long-term-task, long-term-maintenance, short-term-task, and short-term-maintenance. This 2 x 2 matrix is shown in Figure 10-1.

Figure 10-1 Goal Definition Matrix

	TASK	MAINTENANCE
LONG-TERM		
SHORT-TERM		

At this step of the exercise discussion is directed only at clarifying the goal statements and reaching consensus on whether the goal is primarily long or short term and task-related or maintenance-related. Team members should not evaluate the goals at this point, or worry about goal priorities or goal conflicts.

4. The first phase of the exercise has revealed the pattern of goals as viewed by the team. Whether or not the pattern that has emerged is what the team expected is a question that should be discussed.

Phase Two

5. Team members are given a list of all the goal statements in each of the four categories. The team now has an opportunity to correct any errors in the initial sorting.

6. Taking one category at a time, the team is asked to review each statement in the category and eliminate any redundant statements or incorporate them into similar statements. Since there are likely to be a number of duplicate statements, this step should yield four considerably shorter lists.

7. The team is now ready to establish priorities by arranging the remaining goal statements in rank order of importance. Although this can be done numerically (by combining the rank order given to each goal by each participant), it is preferable to arrive at a team consensus through discussion.

This goal setting exercise provides a structured way for the team to share perceptions about goals and priorities. Goal conflicts quickly come out into the open and can at least be discussed, if not resolved. The specific steps of the exercise are less important than its use as a mechanism for the process of team interaction and consensus.

TEAM INTERACTION

Many of the barriers to team effectiveness seem to stem directly from the interaction within the team. The authors in a critical incident study of "ineffective team functioning," found that of 145 incidents reported by 45 health professionals, almost 62 percent were concerned with team problems arising from lack of communication or interprofessional conflict. Often team performance can be improved by alleviating such problems.

Communication Barriers

We have explored in Chapter Seven some of the important aspects of communication among team members. It is important to keep in mind that verbal interaction is only one aspect of team communication, and that among the factors that produce barriers to communication are the following four.

Time. The busy team member often finds there is too little time available for full communication. This is a problem not only in team meetings but also in the informal exchanges of information that take place in the halls or at the nurses' station. If the team approach is to operate effectively, there must be sufficient time to share critical information about patients. It may be necessary to reexamine the advantages of face-to-face interaction versus other means of communication. For example, less time may be required for team meetings if the team makes use of fuller written reports; however, long reports run the risk of not being read at all.

Space. Physical location itself can stimulate or create barriers to free and open communication. The psychologist and social worker whose offices are adjacent to one another are likely to communicate much more frequently than team members who have offices on different floors or in different buildings. Often relocation works to increase the exchange of information among team members, however simply moving offices around does not guarantee increased communication.

Media. Communication may be enhanced by improved recordkeeping systems. The Problem Oriented Medical Record (POMR) seems to have been adopted in many instances as a supplement to the team approach. By focusing on *patient problems* rather than on *a professional discipline,* the system is designed to increase communication among the various professionals working to provide services to a particular client. However, written communication can often be improved without instituting a whole new system of record keeping. Sometimes simply attending more closely to existing records will enhance communication. For example, team members at one agency complained that the physician in charge had sent a patient home over the weekend, but failed to notify the team so that considerable time was spent trying to locate the patient.

Language. Interprofessional differences are sometimes amplified by the use of professional jargon. If team members are speaking different languages, communication will certainly be hindered. Once the problem is recognized, team members can take pains to explain the technical terms they use, checking with other team members to be sure they are communicating clearly. Unfortunately, professional jargon is sometimes used as a symbol of status and expertise, and some professionals hesitate to explain their jargon as though sharing it implied a loss of their unique skills and knowledge. This attitude is often seen in the interaction of professionals and nonprofessionals on the team. Too often the professional conveys a sense of "You really can't understand what I am saying because you don't have sufficient training to comprehend these professional concepts." This does little to encourage effective sharing of information.

There are, of course, still other factors that can enhance or hinder communication within the team, and several of these were discussed in Chapter Seven. A team which is interested in improving its communication patterns may want to address these questions:

- What are the formal and informal channels of communication in this team? Is the communication network one that adequately serves the needs of the team?
- Is sufficient time available to team members for adequate communication? Do physical arrangements enhance communication?
- Do the present record keeping systems enhance communication?

So long as the interdisciplinary team is composed of persons rather than machines or computers, there will be conflicts among team members. An appropriate team goal then is not to eliminate conflict, but to minimize its negative effects.

Conflict Management

A number of the conflict management techniques described in the literature (Robbins, 1974; Blake, Shepard and Morton, 1964; Burke, 1969; Vogt and Ducanis, 1977) are applicable to team conflict situations.

The initial reaction to interpersonal conflict is often to *smooth over* differences and avoid any overt disagreements. This is seldom an adequate solution to the problem. While there may be some temporary relief, it is likely that the conflict will emerge again, perhaps in a more virulent form.

Another approach often employed in dealing with team conflict is *compromise and bargaining*. Unfortunately, this may result in outcomes that satisfy neither party, so resentments continue. An *authoritarian* approach, whereby the team leader enforces a resolution to the conflict, may also do nothing to quell resentments. A more promising approach is to use *problem solving* to reach a rational solution that is satisfactory to all parties. The particular problem-solving techniques used will vary with the nature and extent of the conflict, but generally will involve: (a) identifying the conflict (problem identification), (b) exploring solutions, (c) trying out one of the solutions, and (d) evaluating the solution.

Reducing Role Conflict

A common source of conflict among team members involves ambiguous and overlapping roles. This issue has been addressed at several points in this book because it is such a pervasive problem for interdisciplinary teams.

In part, role ambiguity and role confusion arise because team members are filling several different *kinds* of roles simultaneously. These include:

- *personal roles* — based on individual attributes, such as personality factors
- *professional roles* — based on professional competencies
- *team roles* — based on team interaction and including such roles as leader, follower, mediator, etc.

Team members may respond to any of these multiple roles, and while there may be some correlation between roles (for example, personal roles are often related to team roles), sometimes this is not the case.

The greatest problems for the interdisciplinary team seem to come from the conflicts around professional roles resulting from overlapping responsibilities and competencies. The following steps provide a framework for addressing issues of role conflict.

1. **Clarify role perceptions and expectations.** This can be done through verbal discussion or by writing statements on 3 × 5 cards, as in the goal definition exercise. In either case, each team member should indicate his or her perceptions of the role of each other member.

2. **Identify professional competencies.** Now members have an opportunity to indicate their competencies and explain more fully what their professional responsibilities entail. Often it is difficult for team members to ask each other about their skills or knowledge. This step provides a mechanism for eliciting such information without acknowledging ignorance.

3. **Examine overlapping roles.** Base the discussion on information provided in Step 1 and Step 2.

4. **Renegotiate role assignments.** Negotiation is much easier once there is a better understanding of other members' expectations and competencies.

THE FUTURE OF THE TEAM APPROACH

It is often easy to lose sight of the primary purpose of the team and become involved with organizational structure, interpersonal and interprofessional relationships, team development, and a myriad of other aspects that are characteristic of the system.

But it should be remembered that the interdisciplinary team in human service organizations owes its existence to the need for coordinated care of the client. The team, therefore, should always be focused on the central issue of client care.

What will be the future of the team approach? There is at present no way to answer that question with certainty. However, it is highly probable that *teamwork* is likely to become *more* important in the years ahead. The movement toward specialization will accelerate, and the knowledge base of the professions will continue to expand (perhaps at a somewhat slower rate than in the immediate past). And increasing specialization means a continuing need for coordination, if the client is to receive high-quality care. Thus to avoid the problems inherent in the fragmentation of client services, some form of team approach will be demanded.

References

Ackerly, S. The clinic team. *American Journal of Orthopsychiatry*, 1947, *17*, 191-195.

Allen, K.E., Holm, V.A., & Schiefelbusch, R.L. (Eds.). *Early intervention: A team approach.* Baltimore: University Park Press, 1978.

Allied medical education directory (6th ed.). Chicago: American Medical Association, 1976.

Alperson, B.L. A Boolean analysis of interpersonal perception. *Human Relations*, 1975, *28*, 7, 627-652.

American Association for Respiratory Therapy. *Code of Ethics.* Dallas: A.A.R.T. (no date)

American Dental Association, *Principles of Ethics.* Chicago: A.D.A., 1976.

American Medical Association. Principles of medical ethics. *Opinions and Reports of the Judicial Council.* Chicago: A.M.A., 1971.

American Medical Technologists. *Code of ethics.* A.M.T. (no date).

American Psychological Association. *Ethical standards of psychologists.* Washington, D.C.: A.P.A., 1977.

Anderson, S.B., & Ball, S. *The profession and practice of program evaluation.* San Francisco: Jossey-Bass, 1978.

Anderson, S.B., Ball, S., & Murphy, R.T., & associates. *Encyclopedia of educational evaluation.* Washington, D.C.: Jossey-Bass, 1975.

Aradine, C., & Hansen, M.F. Interdisciplinary teamwork in family health care. *Nursing Clinics of North America*, 1970, *5*, 2, 211-222.

Argyris, C. The incompleteness of social psychological theory: Examples from small group, cognitive consistency, and attribution research. *American Psychologist*, 1969, *24*, 893-908.

Bales, R.F. A set of categories for the analysis of small group interaction. *American Sociological Review*, 1950, *15*, 257-263 (b).

Bales, R.F. How people interact in conferences. *Scientific American*, 1955, *192*, 3, 31-35.

Bales, R.F. *Interaction process analysis: A method for the study of small groups.* Cambridge, Mass.: Addison-Wesley, 1950 (a).

Bales, R.F., & Slater, P. Role differentiation in small decision-making groups. In T. Parsons and R. Bales (Eds.), *Family socialization, and interaction process.* Glencoe, Ill.: Free Press, 1955.

Banta, H.D., & Fox, R.C. Role strains of a health care team in a poverty community. *Social Science and Medicine*, 1972, *6*, 697-722.

Barker, L.M. Specialists and general practitioner in relation to teamwork in medical practice. *Journal of the American Medical Association*, 1922, *78* (March), 76.

Bartlett, H.M. *The participation of medical social workers in the teaching of medical students.* Chicago: American Association of Medical Social Workers, 1939.

Bates, J.E., Lieberman, H., & Powell, R.N. Provisions for health care in the ghetto: The family health team. *American Journal of Public Health,* 1970, *60,* 7, 1222-1224.

Bateson, N. Familiarization, group discussion and risk-taking. *Journal of Experimental Social Psychology,* 1966, *2,* 119-129.

Bavelas, A. A mathematical model for group structures. *Applied Anthropology,* 1948, *7,* 16-30.

Beard, G. Foundations for growth. *The Physical Therapy Review,* 1961, *41,* 843-861.

Beck, H.L. The advantages of a multi-purpose clinic for the mentally retarded. *American Journal of Mental Deficiency,* 1962, *66,* 789-794.

Becker, H.S. The nature of a profession. In H. Nelson (Ed.) *Education for the professions* (Part 2). Chicago: University of Chicago Press, 1962.

Beckhard, R. Organizational implications of team building: The larger picture. In H. Wise, R. Beckhard, I. Rubin, & A.L. Kyte (Eds.) *Making health teams work.* Cambridge, Mass.: Ballinger, 1974.

Bem, D.J., Wallach, M.A., & Kogan, N. Group decision-making under risk of aversive consequences. *Journal of Personality and Social Psychology,* 1965, *1,* 453-460.

Benne, K.D., & Sheats, P. Functional roles of group members. *Journal of Social Issues,* 1948, *4,* 41-49.

Blake, R., Shepard, H., & Morton, J. *Managing intergroup conflict in industry.* Houston: Gulf Publishing Company, 1964.

Blank, A. Effects of group and individual conditions on choice behavior. *Journal of Personality and Social Psychology,* 1968, *8,* 294-298.

Brown, J.A. Toward predicting and managing conflict on the anesthesia care team. *Journal of the American Association of Nurse Anesthetists,* 1977, Feb., 37-42.

Brown, R. *Social psychology.* New York: Free Press, 1965.

Bucher, R. & Strauss, A. Professions in process. *American Journal of Sociology,* 1961, *66,* 325-344.

Bufford, J.I., & Kindig, D. Institute for team development — The next two years. In H. Wise, R. Beckhard, I. Rubin, & A.L. Kyte (Eds.) *Making health teams work.* Cambridge, Mass.: Ballinger, 1974.

Burke, R.J. Methods of resolving interpersonal conflict. *Personnel Administration,* 1969, *32,* 48.

Carlins, E.B., & Raven, B.H. Group structure: Attraction, coalitions, communication, and power. In G. Lindzey & E. Aronson (Eds.) *Handbook of social psychology,* Vol. 4. Reading, Mass.: Addison-Wesley, 1969, 102-204.

Carter, L. On defining leadership. In M. Shiref & M.D. Wilson (Eds.) *Group relations at the crossroads.* New York: Harper and Row, 1953, 262-265.

Cartwright, D. The nature of group cohesiveness. In D. Cartwright & A. Zander (Eds.) *Group dynamics: Research and theory* (3rd edition). New York: Harper and Row, 1968, 91-109.

Cartwright, D., & Zander, A. (Eds.). *Group dynamics: Research and theory* (3rd edition). New York: Harper and Row, 1968.

Caudill, W. *The psychiatric hospital as a small society.* Cambridge, Mass.: Harvard University Press, 1958.

Challela, M. The interdisciplinary team: A role definition in nursing. *Image,* 1979, *11,* 1, 9-15.

Christie, D., & Lawrence, L. Patients and hospitals: A study of the attitudes of stroke patients. *Social Science and Medicine,* 1978, *12,* 49-51.

Clement, D.E., & Schiereck, J.J., Jr. Sex composition and group performance in a visual signal detection task. *Memory and Cognition*, 1973, *1*, 251-255.

Coe, R. *Sociology of medicine*. New York: McGraw-Hill, 1970.

Cogan, M.L. Toward a definition of a profession. *Harvard Educational Review*, 1953, *23*, 33-50.

Connelly, T. *Center for interdisciplinary education in allied health, Summary progress report for the first two years and plans for 1978-79*. University of Kentucky, Lexington, Kentucky, 1978, mimeo.

Coser, R. A home away from home. *Social Problems*, 1956, *4*, 3-17.

Craig, J.W. Teamwork in dentistry. *British Dental Journal*, 1970, Feb. 17, 198-202.

Crisler, J., & Settles, R. An integrated rehabilitation team effort in providing services for multi-disability clients. *Journal of Rehabilitation*, 1979, *45*, 1, 34-38.

Croog, S., & Ver Steeg, D. The hospital as a social system. In H. Freeman, S. Levine, & L. Reeder (Eds.) *Handbook of medical sociology* (2nd edition). Englewood Cliffs: Prentice-Hall, 1972.

Deming, W.E. The logic of evaluation. In M. Guttentag & E.L. Struning (Eds.) *Handbook of evaluation research*, Vol. I. Beverly Hills: Sage Publications, 1975, 53-68.

Devitt, G.A. Commonalities of curricular objectives in the preparation of nurses, physical therapists, occupational therapists, and therapeutic dieticians at the baccalaureate level. Doctoral dissertation, University of Pittsburgh, 1970.

Dion, K.L., Baron, R.S., & Miller, N. Why do groups make riskier decisions than individuals? In L. Berkowitz (Ed.) *Advances in social psychology*, Vol. 5. New York: Academic Press, 1970, 305-377.

Dion, K.L., Miller, N., & Magnon, M.A. Group cohesiveness and social responsibility as determinants of the risky shift. Paper presented at the American Psychological Association meeting, Miami, Florida, September, 1970.

Drew, A.L. Teamwork and total patient care. *Journal of Psychiatric Social Work*, 1953, *23*, 25-31.

Drucker, P.F. Managing the "third sector." *Wall Street Journal*, Oct. 3, 1978.

Ducanis, A.J., & Golin, A.K. Interprofessional perceptions in the interdisciplinary health care team. Paper presented at the meeting of the Association of Schools of the Allied Health Professions, Miami, Florida, November, 1978.

Erikson, E. *Childhood and society* (2nd edition). New York: Norton & Company, 1963.

Fenton, K., Yoshida, R., Maxwell, J., & Kaufman, M. Recognition of team goals: An essential step toward rational decision making. *Exceptional Children*, 1979, *45*, 8, 638-644.

Ferguson, D.A., & Vidmar, N. Familiarization-induced risky and cautious shifts: A replication of sorts. Paper presented at the Midwestern Psychological Association meeting, Cincinnati, Ohio, 1970.

Fiedler, F.E. Personality and situational determinants of leadership effectiveness. In D. Cartwright & A. Zander (Eds.) *Group dynamics: Research and theory* (3rd edition). New York: Harper and Row, 1968, 362-380.

Flanders, J.P., & Thistlethwaite, D.L. Effects of familiarization and group discussion upon risk taking. *Journal of Personality and Social Psychology*, 1967, *5*, 91-97.

Flanders, N.A. *Analyzing teaching behavior*. Reading, Mass.: Addison-Wesley, 1970.

Flanders, N.A. Teacher influence in the classroom. In E.J. Amidon & J.B. Hough (Eds.) *Interaction analysis: Theory research and application*. Reading, Mass.: Addison-Wesley, 1967.

Flexner, A. Is social work a profession? In *Proceedings of the National Conference on Charities and Corrections*. Chicago: Hildemann Printing Company, 1915.

Frank, L.K. Interprofessional communication. *American Journal of Public Health*, 1961, *51*, 1798-1804.

Freidson, E. *Patients' views of medical practice*. New York: Russell Sage Foundation, 1961.

French, J.R.P., Jr. & Raven, B. The bases of social power. In D. Cartwright (Ed.) *Studies in social power*. Ann Arbor, Michigan: Institute for Social Research, 1959, 150-167.

Fry, R.E., Lech, B.A., and Rubin, I. Working with the Primary Care Team. In H. Wise, R. Beckhard, I. Rubin, and A.L. Kyte (Eds.) *Making Health Teams Work*. Cambridge, Mass.: Ballinger, 1974.

Gallagher, E.B. Lines of reconstruction and extension in the Parsonian sociology of illness. *Social Science and Medicine*, 1976, *10*, 207-218.

Gamson, W.A. A theory of coalition formation. *American Sociological Review*, 1961, *26*, 373-382.

Geigle-Bentz, F.L. Communication, democracy, leadership, roles and the team in the interdisciplinary health team approach. Unpublished doctoral dissertation, University of Pittsburgh, 1975.

Gibb, C.A. Leadership. In G. Lindzey & E. Aronson (Eds.) *The handbook of social psychology* (Rev. edition), Vol. 4. Reading, Mass: Addison-Wesley, 1969, 205-282.

Goldman, M. A comparison of individual and group performance for varying combinations of initial ability. *Journal of Personality and Social Psychology*, 1965, *1*, 210-216.

Golin, A.K., & Ducanis, A.J. Interdisciplinary implications of the ethical standards of the health professions. Paper presented at the meeting of the Association of Schools of the Allied Health Professions, Dallas, November, 1977.

Goode, W.J. Encroachment, charlatanism and the emerging profession: Psychology, sociology and medicine. *American Sociological Review*, 1960, *25*, 902-914.

Gordon, G. *Role theory and illness*. New Haven, Conn.: College & University Press, 1966.

Greenwood, E. Attributes of a profession. *Social Work*, 1957, *2*, 3, 44-55.

Guttentag, M., & Struening, E.L. (Eds.) *Handbook of evaluation research*. Beverly Hills: Sage Publications, 1975.

Hackman, J.R. Group influence on individuals. In M.D. Dunnette (Ed.) *Handbook of industrial and organizational psychology*. Chicago: Rand McNally, 1975.

Hackman, J.R., & Morris, C.G. Group tasks, group interaction process, and group performance effectiveness: A review and proposed integration. In L. Berkowitz (Ed.) *Advances in social psychology*. New York: Academic Press, 1975.

Halstead, L.S. Team care in chronic illness: A review of the literature of the past 25 years. *Archives of Physical and Medical Rehabilitation*. November, 1976, *57*, 507-511.

Hare, A.P. *Handbook of small group research* (2nd edition). New York: Free Press, 1976.

Harris, J., Saunders, D., & Zasorin-Connors. A training program for interprofessional health care teams. *Health and Social Work*, 1978, *3*, 36-53.

Hart, V. The use of many disciplines with severely and profoundly handicapped. In E. Sontag, J. Smith, & N. Certo (Eds.) *Educational programming for the severely and profoundly handicapped*. C.E.C. Division on Mental Retardation, 1976.

Haselkorn, F. Some dynamic aspects of interpersonal practice in rehabilitation. *Social Casework*, 1958, *39*, 396-400.

Heilman, M.E. Identification of certain competencies needed by health care personnel in order to function as a health care team. Unpublished doctoral dissertation, University of Pittsburgh, 1977.

Hirschowitz, R.G. Grand rounds circus. *Social Policy*, November/December 1972-January/February 1973, 50-55.

Hoffman, L.R. Homogeneity of member personality and its effect on group problem-solving. *Journal of Abnormal and Social Psychology*, 1959, *58*, 27-32.

Hoffman, L.R., & Maier, N.R.F. Quality and acceptance of problem solutions by members of homogeneous and heterogeneous groups. *Journal of Abnormal and Social Psychology*, 1961, *62*, 401-407.

Hollander, E. Conformity, status and idiosyncrasy credit. *Psychological Review*, 1958, *65*, 117-127.

Holm, V.A. Team issues. In K. Allen, V.A. Holm, & R. Schiefelbusch (Eds.) *Early intervention: A team approach*. Baltimore: University Park Press, 1978, 99-115.

Horwitz, J. Dimensions of rehabilitation teamwork. *Rehabilitation Record*, 1969, *10*, 36-39.

Horwitz, J. *Team practice and the specialist: An introduction to interdisciplinary teamwork*. Springfield, Illinois: Charles Thomas, 1970.

Hudson, J.I., & Giacalone, J.J. Current issues in primary care education: Review and commentary. *Journal of Medical Education*, 1975, *50*, 12, 211-233.

Hughes, E.C. Professions. In K.S. Lynn (Ed.) *The professions in America*. Boston: Houghton Mifflin, 1965.

Hurwitz, J.I., Zander, A.F., & Hymovitch, B. Some effects of power on the relations among group members. In D. Cartwright & A. Zander (Eds.) *Group dynamics: Research and theory*. Evanston, Illinois: Harper and Row, 1968, 291-297.

Hutt, M.L., Menninger, W.C., & O'Keefe, D.E. The neuropsychiatric team in the United States Army. *Mental Health*, 1947, *31*, 103-119.

Infante, M.S., Speranza, K.A., & Gillespie, P.W. An interdisciplinary approach to the education of health professional students. *Journal of Allied Health*, 1976, *5*, 13-22.

Jacobson, S.R. A study of interprofessional collaboration. *Nursing Outlook*, 1974, *22*, 751-755.

Jacques, M. *Rehabilitation counseling: Scope and services*. Boston: Houghton Mifflin, 1970.

Johnson, E.A. Giving the consumer a voice in the hospital business. *Hospital Administration*, 1970, *15*.

Johnson, G.R. The research domain of physical therapy. Unpublished doctoral dissertation, University of Pittsburgh, 1971.

Kelley, H.H., & Thibaut, J.W. Group problem solving. In G. Lindzey & E. Aronson (Eds.) *Handbook of social psychology* (Rev. edition), Vol. 4. Reading, Mass.: Addison-Wesley, 1969, 1-104.

Kindig, D.A. Interdisciplinary education development for primary health care team delivery. *Journal of Medical Education*, 1975, *50*, 97-110.

Kingdon, D.R. *Matrix organization: Managing information technologies*. London: Tavistock, 1973.

Kogan, N., & Wallach, M.A. *Risk-taking: A study in cognition and personality*. New York: Holt, 1964.

Krech, D., & Crutchfield, R.S. *Theory and problems of social psychology*. New York: McGraw-Hill, 1948.

Lacks, P., Landsbaum, J., & Stern, M. Workshop in communication for members of a psychiatric team. *Psychological Reports*, 1970, *26*, 423-430.

Laing, R.D., Phillipson, H., & Lee, A.R. *Interpersonal perception: A theory and a method of research*. New York: Harper and Row, 1966.

Lashof, J.C. The health care team in the mile square area, Chicago. *Bulletin New York Academy of Medicine*, 1968, *44*, 1, 1363-1369.

Laughlin, P.R., Branch, L.G., & Johnson, H.H. Individual versus triadic performance on a unidimensional complementary task as a function of initial ability level. *Journal of Personality and Social Psychology*, 1969, *12*, 144-150.

Leff, W.F., Raven, B.H., & Gunn, R.L. A preliminary investigation of social influence in the mental health professions. *American Psychologist*, 1964, *19*, 505 (abstract).

Levine, S., & White, P.E. The community of health organizations. In H. Freeman, S. Levine, & L. Reeder (Eds.) *Handbook of medical sociology* (2nd edition). Englewood Cliffs: Prentice-Hall, 1972.

Lewis, C., & Resnick, B. Relative orientations of students of medicine and nursing to ambulatory patient care. *Journal of Medical Education*, 1966, *41*, 162-166.

Lieb, J., Lipsitch, I., & Slaby, A. *The crisis team: A handbook for the mental health professional.* Hagerstown, Maryland: Harper and Row, 1973.

Lorber, J. Good patients and problem patients: Conformity and deviance in a general hospital. *Journal of Health and Social Behavior*, 1975, *16*, 213-225.

Marquis, D.G. Individual responsibility and group decisions involving risk. *Industrial Management Review*, 1962, *3*, 8-23.

Martin, H. (Ed.). *The abused child: A multidisciplinary approach to development issues and treatment.* Cambridge, Mass.: Ballinger, 1976.

Mechanic, D., & Volkhart, E.H. Stress, illness behavior and the sick role. *American Sociological Review*, 1961, *26*, 51-58.

Meehl, P.E. *Clinical versus statistical prediction.* Minneapolis: University of Minnesota Press, 1954.

Melia, K. Teamwork eases long-term care admissions. *Hospital Progress*, July, 1978.

Myers, D.G. Enhancement of initial risk-taking tendencies in social situations. Unpublished doctoral dissertation, University of Iowa, 1967.

Myers, D., & Lamm, H. The group polarization phenomenon. *Psychological Bulletin*, 1976, *83*, 4, 602-627.

Nagi, S.Z. Team work in health care in the United States: A sociological perspective. *The Milbank Memorial Fund Quarterly*, Health & Society, 1975, *53*, 75-91.

National Association of Social Workers. *Code of ethics.* Washington, D.C.: N.A.S.W., 1967.

National Rehabilitation Counseling Association. *Ethical standards for rehabilitation counselors.* N.R.C.A., 1972.

Nicolais, J.P. Policy development and strategy in the licensure of speech pathologists and audiologists. *American Journal of Occupational Therapy*, 1976, *30*, 20-26.

Noll, V.H. *Introduction to educational measurement* (2nd edition). Boston: Houghton Mifflin, 1965.

Ort, R.S., Ford, A.B., & Liske, R.E. The doctor-patient relationship as described by physicians and medical students. *Journal of Health and Human Behavior*, 1974, *5*, 25-34.

Parker, A.W. *The team approach to primary health care.* Neighborhood Health Center Seminar Program, monograph series no. 3. California: University Extension, Berkeley, 1972.

Parsons, T. The sick role and the role of the physician reconsidered. *The Milbank Memorial Fund Quarterly*, Health & Society, Summer, 1975, 257-278.

Parsons, T. *The social system.* Glencoe, Ill.: Free Press, 1951.

Parsons, T. Some problems confronting sociology as a profession. *American Sociological Review*, 1959, *24*, 547-559.

Parsons, T. & Fox, R. Therapy and the modern urban family. *Journal of Social Issues*, 1952, *8*, 31-44.

Pascasio, A. Education for the physical therapist of the future. Doctoral dissertation, University of Pittsburgh, 1966.

Patterson, C.H. Is the team concept obsolete? *Journal of Rehabilitation*, 1959, *25*, 2, 9-10; 27-28.

Perrow, C. The analysis of goals in complex organizations. *American Sociological Review*, 1961, *26*, 854-866.

Perrow, C. Goals and power structure. In E. Freidson (Ed.) *The hospital in modern society.* New York: Free Press, 1963.

Pomrinse, S.D. To what degree are hospitals publicly accountable? *Hospitals*, 1969, *43*, 69-74.

Pruitt, D.G., & Teger, A.I. Is there a shift toward risk in group discussion? If so is it a group phenomena? If so, what causes it? Paper presented at the meeting of the American Psychological Association, Washington, D.C., 1967.

Pruitt, D.G., & Teger, A.I. The risky-shift in group betting. *Journal of Experimental Social Psychology*, 1969, *5*, 115-126.

Rae-Grant, Q.A., & Marcuse, D. The hazards of teamwork. *American Journal of Orthopsychiatry*, 1968, *38*, 4-8.

Reitan, H.T., & Shaw, M.E. Group membership, sex-composition of the group, and conformity behavior. *Journal of Social Psychology*, 1964, *64*, 45-51.

Robbins, S. *Managing organizational conflict*. Englewood Cliffs: Prentice-Hall, 1974.

Rocereto, L. *Interschool community project report for students in the health professions*, Part I. University of Pittsburgh, Pittsburgh, Pennsylvania, 1977.

Rogers, C.R. *Client-centered therapy – Its current practice, implications, and theory*. New York: Houghton Mifflin, 1951.

Rubin, I., & Beckhard, R. Factors influencing the effectiveness of health teams. *Milbank Memorial Quarterly*, 1972, *1*, 3, 317-335.

Rubin, I., Plovnick, M., & Fry, R. *Improving the coordination of care: A program for health team development*. Cambridge, Mass: Ballinger, 1975.

Scheff, T.J. Decision rules, types of error, and their consequence in medical diagnosis. *Behavioral Sciences*, 1963, *8*.

Schmitt, B.D. (Ed.). *The child protection team handbook*. New York: Garland STPM Press, 1978.

Scriven, M. The methodology of evaluation. In *Perspectives of curriculum evaluation*. AERA monograph series on Curriculum Evaluation, No. 1. Evanston: Rand McNally, 1967, 39-82.

Segall, A. The sick role concept: Understanding illness behavior. *Journal of Health and Social Behavior*, 1976, *17*, 163-170.

Sells, C., & West, M. Interdisciplinary clinics for the developmentally disabled — Washington State's experience. *Mental Retardation*, October 1976, 19-21.

Shaw, M. Communication networks. In L. Berkowitz (Ed.) *Advances in experimental social psychology*, Vol. 1. New York: Academic Press, 1964.

Shaw, M.E. *Group dynamics: The psychology of small group behavior* (2nd edition). New York: McGraw-Hill, 1976.

Sifneos, P.E. The interdisciplinary team. *Psychiatric Quarterly*, 1969, *43*, 123-129.

Steen, L.A. Computer chess: Mind versus machine. *Science News*, November 29, 1975, *108*, 345-350.

Steiner, I.D. *Group process and productivity*. New York: Academic Press, 1972.

Stoner, J.A.F. A comparison of individual and group decisions involving risk. Unpublished masters thesis. School of Industrial Management: Massachusetts Institute of Technology, 1961.

Stueks, A.M. Working together collaboratively with other professions. *Community Mental Health Journal*, 1965, *1*, 4, 316-319.

Suchman, E.A. Stages of illness and medical care. *Journal of Health and Human Behavior*, 1965, *6*, 114-128.

Sundberg, N.D., & Tyler, L.E. *Clinical psychology*. New York: Appleton-Century-Crofts, 1962.

Sussman, M.B. Occupational sociology and rehabilitation. In M.B. Sussman (Ed.) *Sociology and rehabilitation*. Washington, D.C.: American Sociological Association, 1966.

Szasz, G. Educating for the health team. *Canadian Journal of Public Health*, September/October 1970, 386-390.

Szasz, T., & Hollender, M. A contribution to the philosophy of medicine: The basic models of the doctor-patient relationship. *Archives of Internal Medicine,* 1956, *97,* 585-592.

Tagliacozzo, D., & Mauksch, H. The patient's view of the patient's role. In E. Jaco (Ed.) *Patients, physicians and illness: A source book in behavioral science and health.* New York: Free Press, 1972.

Teger, A.I., & Pruitt, D.G. Components of group risk-taking. *Journal of Experimental Social Psychology,* 1967, *3,* 189-205.

Thibaut, J.W., & Kelley, H.H. *The social psychology of groups.* New York: Wiley, 1959.

Thomas, H. The dynamics of the interdisciplinary team in the adult correctional process. *The Prison Journal,* 1964, *44,* 21-27.

Tichy, M. *Behavioral science techniques: An annotated bibliography for health professionals.* New York: Praeger Publishers, 1975.

Tichy, M. *Health care teams: An annotated bibliography.* New York: Praeger Publishers, 1974.

Tichy, N. *Organizational design for primary health care.* New York: Praeger Publishers, 1977.

Treiman, D.J. *Occupational prestige in comparative perspective.* New York: Academic Press, 1977.

Vogel, E.E. The history of physical therapists, U.S. Army. *Physical Therapy,* 1967, *47,* 1015-1025.

Vogt, M., & Ducanis, A. Conflict and cooperation in the allied health professions. *Journal of Allied Health,* 1977, *6,* 1, 23-30.

Vollmer, H.M., & Mills, D.L. (Eds.) *Professionalization.* Englewood Cliffs: Prentice-Hall, 1966.

Wagner, R. Rehabilitation team practice. *Rehabilitation Counseling Bulletin,* 1977, *21,* 2, 206-217.

Walker, H.M., & Lev, J. *Statistical inference.* New York: Henry Holt, 1953.

Wallach, M.A., & Kogan, N. The roles of information, discussion and consensus in group risk-taking. *Journal of Experimental Social Psychology,* 1965, *1,* 1-19.

Wallach, M.A., Kogan, N., & Bem, D.J. Diffusion of responsibility and level of risk taking in groups. *Journal of Abnormal and Social Psychology,* 1964, *68,* 263-274.

Wallach, M.A., Kogan, N., & Burt, R. Can group members recognize the effects of group discussion upon risk-taking? *Journal of Experimental Social Psychology,* 1965, *1,* 379-395.

Webster's third new international dictionary, unabridged. Springfield, Mass.: G. & C. Merriam Company, 1976.

Weiner, D., & Raths, O. Contributions of the mental hygiene clinic team to clinic decisions. *American Journal of Orthopsychiatry,* 1959, *29,* 350-356.

Weinstein, A.S. Evaluation through medical records and related information systems. In M. Guttentag & E.L. Streuning (Eds.) *Handbook of evaluation research,* Vol. 1, Beverly Hills: Sage Publications, 1975, 397-481.

Weisbord, M.R. Why organization development hasn't worked (so far) in medical centers. *Health Care Maintenance Review,* 1976, *1,* 1, 17-28.

Weiss, C. Evaluation research in the political context. In M. Guttentag & E.L. Streuning (Eds.) *Handbook of evaluation research,* Vol. 1. Beverly Hills: Sage Publications, 1975, 13-26.

Weitz, H. *Behavior change through guidance.* New York: Wiley & Sons, 1964.

Wendland, C.J., & Crawford, C.C. *Team delivery of primary health care.* Los Angeles County Medical Training System, 1976.

Whitehouse, F.A. Teamwork — A democracy of professions. *Exceptional Children,* 1951, *18,* 5-52.

Wile, E. The team approach in a rehabilitation agency for the blind. *The New Outlook,* 1970, *64,* 2, 33-37.

Wilson, A.J. Teamwork conference yields high dividends. *Journal of Rehabilitation*, 1962, *28*, 2, 23-25.

Wilson, R. The physician's changing hospital role. *Human Organization*, 1959, *18*, 177-183.

Wilson, R. The social structure of a general hospital. *Annals of the American Academy of Political and Social Science*, 1963, *346*, 67-76.

Wilson, R. *The sociology of health.* New York: Random House, 1970.

Wilson, R., & Bloom, S. Patient-practitioner relationships. In H. Freeman, S. Levine, & L. Reeder (Eds.) *Handbook of medical sociology* (2nd edition). Englewood Cliffs: Prentice-Hall, 1972.

Winter, M. The rehabilitation team: A catalyst to risky rehabilitation decisions? *Rehabilitation Counseling Bulletin*, 1976, *19*, 4, 581-586.

Wright, B.A. *Physical disability – A psychological approach.* New York: Harper and Row, 1960.

Zander, A., Cohen, A.R., & Stotland, E. Power and relations among professions. In D. Cartwright (Ed.) *Studies in social power.* Ann Arbor, Michigan: Institute for Social Research, 1959, 15-34.

Zola, I.K. Culture and symptoms: An analysis of patients' presenting complaints. *American Sociological Review*, 1966, *31*, 615-630.

Index

NOTE: Italicized numbers indicate figures or tables.

About the Authors

Alex J. Ducanis received his doctorate in educational administration from the University of Pittsburgh where he is now Professor of Higher Education and of the Health Related Professions. His academic interests are in research methodology, the American college and university, and the interdisciplinary team. He has published numerous research and scholarly papers and is a frequent contributor at professional meetings. Before returning to the University of Pittsburgh he served as Director of Institutional Research at the State University of New York at Binghamton and as Educational Research Associate in the New York State Education Department. He also served as the first Director of the Institute for Higher Education at the University of Pittsburgh.

Anne K. Golin received her doctorate in clinical psychology at the University of Iowa. She holds the rank of Professor in the School of Education at the University of Pittsburgh, with a joint appointment in Rehabilitation Counseling and Special Education. Before going to the University of Pittsburgh, Dr. Golin served as a Field Assessment Officer for the Peace Corps Training Program at the University of Wisconsin-Milwaukee. Her primary academic interests are in psychology of exceptional children, psychology of disability, mental health, and the interdisciplinary team. She has presented a number of papers at professional meetings, is a contributor to professional journals in psychology and rehabilitations, and has conducted workshops concerning the interdisciplinary team.